THE
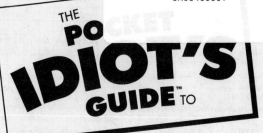
POCKET
IDIOT'S
GUIDE™ TO

Bioidentical Hormones

by Ricki Pollycove, M.D., M.S.
with Nancy Faass, M.S.W., M.P.H.

ALPHA

A member of Penguin Group (USA) Inc.

ALPHA BOOKS

Published by the Penguin Group

Penguin Group (USA) Inc., 375 Hudson Street, New York, New York 10014, USA

Penguin Group (Canada), 90 Eglinton Avenue East, Suite 700, Toronto, Ontario M4P 2Y3, Canada (a division of Pearson Penguin Canada Inc.)

Penguin Books Ltd., 80 Strand, London WC2R 0RL, England

Penguin Ireland, 25 St. Stephen's Green, Dublin 2, Ireland (a division of Penguin Books Ltd.)

Penguin Group (Australia), 250 Camberwell Road, Camberwell, Victoria 3124, Australia (a division of Pearson Australia Group Pty. Ltd.)

Penguin Books India Pvt. Ltd., 11 Community Centre, Panchsheel Park, New Delhi—110 017, India

Penguin Group (NZ), 67 Apollo Drive, Rosedale, North Shore, Auckland 1311, New Zealand (a division of Pearson New Zealand Ltd.)

Penguin Books (South Africa) (Pty.) Ltd., 24 Sturdee Avenue, Rosebank, Johannesburg 2196, South Africa

Penguin Books Ltd., Registered Offices: 80 Strand, London WC2R 0RL, England

International Standard Book Number: 978-1-59257-976-1
Library of Congress Catalog Card Number: 2009934678

12 11 10   8 7 6 5 4 3 2 1

Interpretation of the printing code: The rightmost number of the first series of numbers is the year of the book's printing; the rightmost number of the second series of numbers is the number of the book's printing. For example, a printing code of 10-1 shows that the first printing occurred in 2010.

Printed in the United States of America

Note: This publication contains the opinions and ideas of its author. It is intended to provide helpful and informative material on the subject matter covered. It is sold with the understanding that the author and publisher are not engaged in rendering professional services in the book. If the reader requires personal assistance or advice, a competent professional should be consulted.

The author and publisher specifically disclaim any responsibility for any liability, loss, or risk, personal or otherwise, which is incurred as a consequence, directly or indirectly, of the use and application of any of the contents of this book.

Contents

This book is dedicated to the thousands of women who have entrusted me with their health care and shared their personal stories. I also thank my remarkable daughter, Leah, and my mother, Rosalyn, who have broadened my vision of what it means to be a woman, and added vast amounts of love to my life.

Introduction

For women, estrogen turns out to be the key to healthy aging. But for the past seven years, it has been at the center of a storm of controversy. The goal of this book is to answer important questions raised in this debate, separating fact from fiction. You need to know which hormones are safe hormones, and which aren't. It matters, because when we get it right, estrogen helps us age with grace, energy, and better health.

The bioidenticals are newer, safer hormones that are exact copies of those made in a woman's body, atom for atom. They mirror the design and natural balance of female hormones. Provided in cream, gel, or patch, bioidenticals are absorbed through the skin, much like our own hormones. This has proven to be a safer way to use hormone therapy, without the health risks of earlier products.

What's Inside

This book offers a doctor's insight, told through the stories of individual women. Written in everyday terms, these stories are paired with research from around the world involving millions of women. The numbers speak for themselves: women age better with fewer health problems once estrogen is restored. This vital hormone protects us from heart attacks, strokes, and Alzheimer's. Estrogen also resolves the outrageous symptoms of menopause, which makes for better sleep, better skin, and better sex.

You'll find information you can take to your doctor or health-care provider, so you can work together to make the right decisions for your care.

Here's what you'll find in this book:

Chapter 1 offers the view that for women, estrogen really is the secret to graceful aging—with insight on why this topic is important, how the controversies began, and the real truth about estrogen safety.

Chapter 2 time-travels through the history of traditional hormone therapy, looks at how the first products were developed, and includes pros and cons for their use.

Chapter 3 introduces bioidentical hormones and explains what they are, why they are so much safer, and why many women prefer them to earlier types of hormones. The chapter touches on the research, showing how bioidenticals improve symptoms of estrogen depletion, such as hot flashes, insomnia, and low libido.

Chapter 4 offers suggestions on finding the right doctor—someone local who is attuned to what you want and can monitor your health over time. This chapter delves into issues with mail-order bioidenticals compared with the safer FDA-approved bioidenticals that meet much higher standards.

Chapter 5 is all about working with your care provider to develop your own personal plan, including when to start, which hormones to take, whether to use the pill, patch, cream, or ring, at what dosage, and how to know if it's working for you.

Chapter 6 troubleshoots midlife sleep problems and hot flashes and what can be done about them—and explains how you can use hormones and lifestyle to get a better night's sleep.

Chapter 7 is all about blue moods, explaining why hormone supplements tend to improve mood for about 70 percent of women. The chapter also explores the link between food and mood, how to use exercise to boost optimal brain chemistry, and when to call the doctor for mood issues.

Chapter 8 reveals three of the best-kept secrets of weight loss—why hormones can be crucial in avoiding weight gain, the skinny on *real* "comfort food," and how to find your groove for life-long weight mastery.

Chapter 9 takes a closer look at skin, the deeper effects of low estrogen on our skin, and how hormone supplements help the complexion with effective solutions for lustrous skin.

Chapter 10 gives the good news about sex in midlife and what estrogen can do to restore sizzle to your sexuality and rekindle your relationship.

Chapter 11 tackles the topic of Alzheimer's and explains the tremendous protection that estrogen provides against heart attacks, dementia, Parkinson's, and stroke. These issues come alive when viewed through the true-to-life stories of four women.

Chapter 12 offers insight on maintaining inner balance. The personal stories in this final chapter show how women maintain their gains and sustain their progress at every phase in their life journey.

There are three different sidebars found throughout the book.

def•i•ni•tion

These definitions go beyond the media and the hype to provide you with nuggets of important information.

Warning Label

The Warning Labels bring you information that is easily overlooked, but which turns out to be crucial in making healthy decisions.

Hormone Tips

The Hormone Tips are practical insights gleaned from daily clinical practice that many women have found useful in their own lives.

Acknowledgments

I wish to thank Alpha Books for the opportunity to create this book on a vital life-enhancing and potentially lifesaving subject. Randy Ladenheim-Gil and her insightful professional staff have been exceptional throughout the process. I also want to express my gratitude to Nancy Faass for her superb writing skills and for sustaining the pace and quality necessary to such a detailed timely volume.

Trademarks

All terms mentioned in this book that are known to be or are suspected of being trademarks or service marks have been appropriately capitalized. Alpha Books and Penguin Group (USA) Inc. cannot attest to the accuracy of this information. Use of a term in this book should not be regarded as affecting the validity of any trademark or service mark.

Chapter 1

Hormones—What's New, What's True?

In This Chapter

- What are the realities of "aging naturally"
- Why there are drawbacks to aging without hormone support
- How estrogen protects us against Alzheimer's, strokes, heart attacks, and crumbling bones
- What the truth is about estrogen and cancer
- Why bioidenticals are safer

As an OB/GYN, the first question women usually ask me is, "Do I really need estrogen?" It's appealing to think of aging "naturally." This is especially true after all the bad press that hormones have gotten in the media.

Studies tracking the health of almost a million women have made it clear that healthy aging requires estrogen. Supplementing estrogen is one of the most effective solutions science has found to counter the effects of aging.

The other good news is that hormone products have become much safer, so a woman no longer has to trade one health risk for another. The new bioidentical estrogen and progesterone provide all the benefits of earlier hormone products, without the added risks or side effects.

The Myth of Natural Aging

What is *natural aging*? We imagine the generations of vigorous women who have gone before us— revolutionary war widows, pioneers, farm women, suffragettes, all aging naturally. But the reality turns out to be quite different than you'd expect. At the time of the Revolutionary War, only one American woman in twenty lived to the age of 50 (to experience menopause). The average life expectancy for women was 32.

A century later, in 1900, life expectancy had increased to 50 (for white, American women). That means one woman in two reached the age of 50. In the 1920s, the suffragettes, getting the right to vote for women, took center stage. Looking at the photos of these elderly women, it's a little shocking to realize that most of them were actually in their 40s.

Today, life expectancy for the average American woman is 84. Our life span has been extended through the miracles of science and medicine, paired with public health services and the control of infectious disease. Now that we're living longer, our primary concern becomes healthy aging and quality of life. The Baby Boomer generation is the first group of women to enter menopause with clear expectations for a longer and more engaged life than they observed in their mothers. This is a good time to set the record straight.

Hormone Tips

What is natural menopause? Among all the primates, only the chimpanzee lives more than a few months after her last offspring. In nature, menopause is virtually unknown and unnatural. The human race has enhanced survival with modern medicine and science. We may live longer, for example, because we took antibiotics for a life-threatening infection or took medication to prevent a heart attack or had surgery to survive an accident. Yet after we enter the biologically unnatural state of menopause, we want to "go natural." Why leave all the intelligent advances behind just when the going gets tough?

Healthy Aging Requires Estrogen

Throughout a woman's child-bearing years, her health is supported by her hormones. With menopause, many of those protections are lost. As estrogen levels decline and fertility decreases, these built-in supports are withdrawn. When estrogen levels fall, all women experience major changes in their body chemistry—even those who do not have hot flashes or insomnia. Long-term, the loss of estrogen results in devastating effects, reflected in diseases of aging such as osteoporosis and Alzheimer's.

We used to think that a healthy lifestyle would sustain us through these "golden years." But for the vast majority of women, exercise and a good diet simply aren't enough. Research has shown that estrogen is the key. In my practice, with more than 6,000 patients, less than 10 percent of the women older than 70 are able to retain vigorous good health without hormone supplements.

Despite the best efforts of daily physical activity, yoga, an optimal diet, and vitamin supplements, women who are not taking estrogen experience a steady loss of bone, connective tissue, and muscle after menopause.

The Downside of No HRT

From a doctor's perspective, unless the symptoms of menopause are intrusive, for most women life is pretty good without added estrogen until about 70. Big problems are relatively rare. The real concern is what happens after 75—the little problems with bone and muscle loss, higher blood pressure, and climbing cholesterol start to add up, and life becomes more often fraught with disability. Many women see this firsthand as they care for their elderly mothers.

In the first 10 years of menopause, women find that they are able to avoid the worst symptoms with life-style changes and local creams for vaginal dryness. Yet as estrogen levels continue to fall and remain at very low levels, the ravages of bone loss, shrinking muscle mass, and fractures begin to take their toll on quality of life. Rates of dementia increase with every passing decade. Unfortunately, dementia rates for women significantly exceed those in men. Supplementing estrogen at a minimal level supports better health in all the systems of the body and cuts the risk of dementia by more than a third.

Today the average woman lives 30 years beyond menopause. We see predictable problems develop at every age following menopause:

- After 50—Insomnia, hot flashes, arthritis, and weight gain
- After 60—Continued weight gain and diabetes
- After 70—Increased incidence of deadly heart attacks, stroke, osteoporosis, and fatal hip fractures
- After 80—Significant risk of Alzheimer's and Parkinson's, and loss of independent living

Thirty years is a long time to live without estrogen, so it is important to revisit the decisions about whether to take hormones to support your health long-term. You want to put this thought process on the front burner, early in the game.

Avoiding Alzheimer's

Among the diseases of aging, Alzheimer's is perhaps the most daunting. By age 85, one person in three will develop Alzheimer's. Estrogen, started early in menopause, has been found to be highly protective against this devastating form of dementia.

Estrogen also has protective effects for the brain, heart, bones, muscles, and skin throughout our life span. Unfortunately, the loss of estrogen during menopause removes these protections. Research published in 2007, 2008, and 2009 reports that the earlier a woman loses her hormones, the greater her risk of Alzheimer's and Parkinson's. For these women, dementia and Parkinson's also tend to develop earlier in life.

It's sad to read these reports, because once Alzheimer's is diagnosed, it is really too late. The damage has been done. At present, there is no treatment known to science that will undo the destruction of brain tissue caused by Alzheimer's. But we can certainly lower the risk if we take preventative steps early in menopause. We know that women who use estrogen therapy within the first 10 years of menopause have at least 30 percent less risk of Alzheimer's disease compared with those who do not take estrogen. (The same is true of heart disease.)

What is the hormone connection with mental function? It turns out that every cell in the brain is directly influenced by the presence of estrogen. Maintaining those estrogen levels is key to the health of the mind. Among women who take estrogen and exercise, even more than a third are able to avoid Alzheimer's.

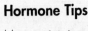

Hormone Tips

Men maintain serum estrogen levels of about 40 pgm/ml from boyhood until they are about 70. Girls share this low level of estrogen until they have their first period. Women's estrogen levels, at the height of their ovulation, average about 500. However, in perimenopause those numbers can range from more than 1,000 to less than 10 pgm/ml. The optimal level of estradiol during supplementation is approximately 30 to 50. This small but crucial level serves to slow the loss of bone and reduces the risk of Alzheimer's and other types of dementia.

Fewer Strokes and Heart Attacks

When estrogen drops, increase in harmful blood fats can occur, such as LDL cholesterol, and tri-glycerides. If your cholesterol rises for a little while, that's no big deal. But when both cholesterol and blood pressure rise, as estrogen levels fall, those events put a woman at greater risk for all kinds of problems. As a result, we see the rates of heart disease increase dramatically after age 60 in women who do not take estrogen.

The hormone connection to heart health is the protective effect of estrogen against inflammation.

Studies on thousands of woman show that supplementing estrogen in the first 10 years of menopause lowers the rate of heart disease by 37 percent.

Preventing Crumbling Bones

What about osteoporosis—bone loss, fractures, broken hip bones, crumbling vertebrae, and height loss?

Low estrogen acts as a signal to literally pull calcium from a woman's bones. This mimics calcium loss during breast feeding, when nature pulls calcium from the mother's bones to provide minerals for the infant. After nursing is over, the body restores these levels. But bone losses after menopause have no built-in mechanism to reverse them, resulting in more osteoporosis unless women take hormones or some form of medication. Think of any woman you know who is older than 70. Chances are she has lost at least a few inches in height, may have poor posture or worse, and has probably suffered a broken vertebra or two. The longer it's been since a woman's menopause, the higher her risk of fracture.

The good news here is that supplementing estrogen prevents 85 percent of osteoporosis. All studies on bone health after age 50 agree and the FDA recognizes estrogen as safe and effective for the prevention of osteoporosis following menopause. It is also encouraging to know that bone loss is actually reversed in women who begin estrogen supplementation.

> **Warning Label**
>
> Osteoporosis after menopause can result in a number of conditions that compromise quality of life. "The widow's hump" we sometimes see in elderly women is an indication that the vertebrae in the spine are collapsing. Crumbling bones can also result in a "fragility fractures" such as a broken hip. Despite the miracles of modern medicine, 25 percent of all hip fractures are still fatal. Fortunately, supplementing with estrogen has been shown to prevent 85 percent of these tragic conditions.

A Short History of HRT

The first estrogen product to appear on the American market was Premarin, approved by the FDA in 1942. Premarin (which is short for *Pre*gnant *Mar*e's Ur*ine*) is derived from the urine of pregnant horses. Throughout the book, we'll refer to this product as Premarin or equine estrogen.

For millions of women this hormone supplement was a God-send, because it provided real relief from the worst symptoms of menopause. For the first time, menopausal women could escape insomnia, hot flashes, mood swings, and depression, and function more normally again. Clearly this was a step forward, especially for women who were really suffering the effects of menopause.

These improvements were not just imaginary. Hundreds of major studies have tracked and confirmed the benefits of Premarin, not only to relieve 95 percent of the symptoms of menopause, but also to help sustain optimal health. Among women who began hormone therapy with equine estrogen before they turned 60, there are clear, undisputed improvements in their health. Premarin has done a good job overall. But with safer products available today, we are likely to do even better.

The Cancer Scares

Initially doctors considered estrogen risk-free—the hormone fountain of youth and the key to staying "feminine forever." The first sign that this might not be true came from alarming research findings published in 1975. Researchers found an increase in uterine cancer among women who took estrogen but did not balance it with progesterone, another important hormone.

Why? In a woman's body, nature does not work through a single hormone alone, but through several hormones acting in concert. Researchers found that using estrogen alone increased the risk of a form of uterine cancer. To reproduce the protective effects of a woman's natural hormone cycles, estrogen must be taken in combination with progesterone.

Because women who have had a hysterectomy no longer have the risk of uterine cancer, they do not require the added progesterone. These women may be prescribed estrogen alone.

Breast Cancer: False Alarm

The next scare to hit the media focused on breast cancer. News reports reflected the same sensationalist style of the first media blockbusters. These findings were based on a study of 16,000 women using Premarin and progestin, taken in the combination product PremPro.

Sometimes science unintentionally becomes a numbers game. Although researchers reported an increase in breast cancer, the actual number of cases of cancer turned out to be exceptionally low. Essentially, eight additional cases were identified per every 10,000 women. To put this in perspective, eating one weekly serving of grapefruit or French fries increases your cancer risk at a rate comparable to PremPro. Using an electric blanket or working as an airline hostess has four times the breast cancer risk of PremPro. But are these just quirks of data collection or do they really mean something?

The 2002 finding was reversed in 2007, with barely a whisper from the media. When the data were reanalyzed, it was reported that there was actually *no* risk at all. Unfortunately, busy doctors and specialists who did not read that article in the medical literature are not aware of this new data. This was really great news, but it did not register in the public mind or serve to lower fears about breast cancer and hormones.

What the study *actually* found that was statistically significant is a 20 percent *lower* risk of breast cancer in the users of estrogen (the product Premarin™)

as compared to women taking the inactive dummy pills (the placebo). Virtually all other research studies published since 2000 are in agreement that estrogen does not cause cancer, but in fact protects women against cancer. This experience makes it clear that no single research study has a corner on the truth.

The media has not helped us overcome these fears. When researchers came out with a new report finding virtually *no* increase in breast cancer *or* heart disease, this good news made much less of a splash. The shadow side of the media industry tends to play on fear as an attention-getter to keep audiences glued to their television.

In the medical community, many doctors continue to be unaware of the reassessment and the new data on estrogen's protective effects against cancer. As a result, most women still believe that estrogen causes breast cancer. Old misconceptions are slow to fade.

Enter Bioidenticals

The search for safer hormone products has continued over the past five decades. The new hormone products reflect advances in physics and technology that were simply not available 60 years ago, when extracts of animal hormones were our only option.

The next generation of hormone products, bioidenticals, are created from plant-based molecules. These hormones have a structure identical to that of human hormones. Bioidenticals begin with yam or soy molecules, which are then restructured in the laboratory to duplicate the chemical composition of human estrogen and other hormones.

Bioidentical hormones are indistinguishable from those made in a woman's body. Their chemical formula has been verified by the most subtle testing available to modern science. These new hormones duplicate the exact chemical structures that nature has road-tested for millions of years, since the first humans.

This formulation offers a number of major safety advantages. Bioidenticals are typically taken through the skin, transdermally, as a patch, gel, spray, or a cream, rather than by mouth. This duplicates the way in which sex hormones are delivered in the body. Our endocrine hormones are absorbed directly into the bloodstream rather than through the digestive tract and the liver.

Transdermals avoid the health issues that can result when hormones are taken in tablet form, by mouth. Hormones taken orally must be processed by the liver, resulting in an increased incidence of blood clots and other related risks. Safety is higher with hormones absorbed through the skin or vagina, rather than by mouth, because they do not cause increased risk of clotting.

Benefits of Estrogen Therapy

Health is the secret to quality of life. The research makes it clear that estrogen supports true quality of life and healthier aging:

- Reduction in heart disease—37 percent
- Fewer bone fractures—30 percent
- Less breast cancer—18 percent
- Less diabetes—12 percent
- Fewer strokes—11 percent
- Longer life—29 percent

Studies conducted over the past 15 years have confirmed the absolute safety of bioidentical estrogen and progesterone, used in combination, and their protective effects against the diseases of aging.

A Short History of Hormones

In This Chapter

- Revealing the difference between bioidentical estrogen and horse estrogen
- Showing why it can be dangerous to take estrogen without progesterone
- Debunking the myth that estrogen causes cancer
- Disclosing the fact that horse estrogens contain more than 400 compounds foreign to a woman's body

A hundred years ago, women with "melancholia" were successfully treated with extracts of animal adrenal glands and testicles. (Freud described this form of treatment in his writings.) Glandular extracts were still used to treat menopause as recently as the 1930s, when the primary hormone therapy available to women continued to be based on testosterone.

The First Estrogens

At that point, we did not yet have the ability to characterize or synthesize hormones in the laboratory, so it's not surprising that the first estrogen product was also derived from animal extracts.

What Is Premarin?

Equine estrogen was the first form of estrogen to be used in hormone products. Extracted from the urine of pregnant mares, this product is marketed under the brand name Premarin. It is also referred to as conjugated estrogen, which describes the paired molecules of horse estrogen that it contains. Premarin provided a more effective treatment for symptom relief than earlier hormone therapies for women using testosterone. In this formulation, mare's urine is collected, the hormones are extracted, purified, and concentrated, and the dosage is standardized. The product is then packed into tablet form, coated with shellac, and packaged for distribution. This hormone supplement continues to be available on the market today and is used by millions of women.

Equine estrogen was one of the first medications released under the FDA's new process of product review. FDA approval, initiated the year before in 1941, provided some means of control over patent medicines, which sometimes delivered a useful remedy and sometimes a toxic brew. The initial FDA guidelines required research on safety and efficacy, and on reliability of production.

How Effective Is It?

Equine estrogen was found to be very effective.
Women suffering the worst symptoms of menopause were those most likely to seek health care
for their symptoms. Of the women who took this
new estrogen for hot flashes, 95 percent found their
symptoms completely relieved to their satisfaction,
often within three months. It was equally useful for
menopausal insomnia, particularly the type of sleep
interruption that occurs in the middle of the night.
Equine estrogen was also terrific for curing vaginal
dryness. However, after about 30 years of use, a
dangerous side effect of the hormone was identified.
At that point, the fear of estrogen began.

The Real Cancer Risk

By 1975, reports of uterine cancer were appearing
in the medical literature and began making head-
lines. The medical community had reached the consensus that equine estrogen significantly increased
the risk of uterine cancer, if given without the com-
panion hormone progesterone to balance it.

One Hormone or Two?

In a woman's body, nature does not work through
a single hormone alone, but through several hormones acting in concert. These elegantly coor-
dinated effects are reflected in every aspect of a
woman's health. In pre-menopausal women, the
monthly cycle consists of the following events.

1. The rise in estrogen, which prompts the release of an egg from the ovaries.
2. The release of progesterone, which prepares the uterine lining for pregnancy, forming a layer of blood-rich tissue to support a developing egg.
3. If conception does not occur, the ovaries stop producing progesterone and this inner layer is shed—this is a woman's monthly menstrual flow.

Progesterone is the chemical messenger that signals a halt to the build-up of the uterine lining. The drop in progesterone level starts this shedding process, cleansing the uterine lining. This process renders the lining thin and healthy at the end of every normal monthly cycle.

Estrogen cues the build-up of the lining, but without *progesterone*, no predictable cleansing process occurs. If estrogen is given without progesterone, "unopposed," the estrogen will continue to stimulate the build-up of this uterine tissue. This can lead to a dangerous thickening of the uterine lining (the endometrium).

Over time the excess build-up of lining tissue in the uterus can become cancerous, resulting in endometrial cancer. Although this form of cancer is very curable when discovered early, it is a very real risk associated with the use of estrogen without *progesterone*.

def•i•ni•tion

Progesterone is a naturally occurring female hormone produced after ovulation, during the second half of the menstrual cycle. Progesterone prepares the uterine lining for pregnancy. When a fertilized egg is implanted, and pregnancy occurs, progesterone helps maintain the pregnancy. Progestins are synthetic hormones that act like progesterone (they're not bioidentical). They were invented to have a suppressive effect on the uterine lining at very low doses. At higher doses, they are a key ingredient in birth control pills.

Rethinking HRT

After the risk of uterine cancer was identified, hormone protocol was rewritten to avoid the build-up of uterine tissue. The standard of care became the use of some form of progesterone, given either the second half of every month (cyclically) or daily in combination with estrogen (continuously).

The first synthetic progesterones were referred to as progestin, with several types still in common usage. (Bioidentical progesterone had not yet been developed.) The most well-known progestin is Medroxyprogesterone Acetate (MPA for short) marketed under the brand name Provera.

- **Cyclical use.** When *progestin (MPA)* is taken 12 to 14 days each month to duplicate a woman's cycle, this is referred to as cyclical use.

- **Continuous use.** When progestin is taken continuously with estrogen, the hormone virtually prevents any growth of the uterine lining, with no expected cycles of bleeding. This type of hormone therapy regimen is described as "continuous combined" hormone replacement therapy. Although this delivery does not mimic the body's natural rhythms, it has been effective in the prevention of endometrial cancer.

Hormone Tips

Taking **progestin (MPA)** 14 days a month duplicates a woman's cycle, so that sounds like the healthiest option, right? But the research shows otherwise. Unless the progestin is included in the same pill as the Premarin, women tend to forget to take it. As a result, the uterine lining does not shed that monthly build-up to keep the uterine wall thin and healthy. This is an example of the interplay between nature, health habits, and long-term consequences.

Data on the use of estrogen and progestin (MPA) in combination from the Women's Health Initiative found a 22 percent reduction in uterine cancer among women on combination hormones, compared with those who used no hormones at all.

As a result of these findings, the vast majority of women who take equine estrogen use it in combination with progestin (MPA). In combination with Premarin, progestin (MPA) is provided in the product PremPro (Premarin plus Provera) in a combination tablet. However, there are some downsides to the use of MPA that will be discussed later in this chapter.

Following Nature's Blueprint

Hormone cycling is basic to the physiology of all menstruating women, so progesterone is also relevant for women taking bioidentical estrogen (estradiol).

Estrogen in all its forms stimulates the uterine lining to greater or lesser degrees. For this reason, women taking bioidenticals also need to take progesterone along with their estrogen, either on a cyclical or continuous basis. There are a few exceptions to this rule, but they are rare.

This safety issue is part of the concern about advertisements posted on the Internet for bioidentical products. From a quick read these ads say there is no risk with natural products. This overlooks the vital importance of giving both estrogen and progesterone in the appropriate form and amount. Gynecologists and family physicians are already seeing an increase in cases of uterine cancer in women taking bioidentical estrogens without adequate progesterone.

As mentioned, for women who have had a hysterectomy, these issues are of no concern at all. They can safely take estrogen alone, and neither progestin nor bioidentical progesterone is needed.

Estrogen Can Be a Lifesaver

Another aspect of the estrogen misunderstanding focuses on the role of estrogen receptors in normal breast tissue and cancerous tissue. This confusion exists not only in the public mind, but also within the medical profession. The answer involves cell biology, membrane chemistry, gene expression, and receptor binding, so it is beyond the scope of this pocket guide.

However, in the simplest terms, the key function of estrogen within each cell is to signal the cell to *stop* growing and to be "well behaved." Cancer cells have an entirely different lifecycle, because their primary danger is uninhibited growth. When cancer is present, estrogen is not the cause of the cancer, but it does bring the cancer to our attention at earlier, more curable stages of development.

Estrogen can literally be a lifesaver when it comes to cancer. Women on hormone therapy have better bloodflow to breast tissue, which is thought to improve rates of early detection.

Impeccable research in the past 20 years has shown that estrogen does not cause breast cancer. However, when tumors do form, we are able to detect these cancers earlier in women using estrogen. For these women, the tumors are detected earlier on mammo-gram imaging. Finding a tumor earlier means it is far more likely to be diagnosed at a stage where it can be removed completely, often without a mastec-tomy.

By bringing these problems to our attention earlier, a woman is much more likely to survive cancer-free and live a healthy, vital, full life. The largest volume of data on breast cancer and estrogen use clearly shows that women on estrogen diagnosed with can-cer have significantly better prognoses, better rates of cure, are less likely to require mastectomy, and do not have higher rates of cell division.

If these facts are at odds with what you know, you are not alone. There is no simple answer to the question of what actually causes breast cancer. Every few weeks there is another study that looks at some factor (being overweight, having a stressful life, etc.) and we shudder in fear again. It cannot be overstated that there is no sleeping dragon that will be awakened by taking estrogen. But if there is an abnormal cell cluster hidden inside the breast, we are most likely to find it earlier in a woman taking estrogen after menopause.

My comments here are based on my experience as a gynecologist, and also as a cancer researcher and a cancer surgeon. By virtue of my medical and scien-tific background, my gynecology practice has always had a significantly greater number of breast cancer survivors. Hundreds of these vitally engaged, thriv-ing women have shared their life stories and health challenges with me over several decades. These experiences are the basis for my commitment to understand and share the truth about breast cancer with women everywhere.

Risks of Oral Hormones

The reports on equine estrogen continue to alternate between good news and bad news. Although the theory of using equine estrogen and progestin (MPA) in combination is sound, these first hormone products have certain limitations. Because equine estrogen is provided by mouth, in tablet form, it can have harmful side effects, increasing the rate of blood clots.

Side Effects

In a woman's body, her own estrogen is gradually released directly into the bloodstream, nourishing every cell and tissue with beneficial effects. Each tiny cell has "machinery" that enables it to respond to estrogen. The liver also gets in on the act, but it's not the primary gateway for estrogen processing. The main route of transmission is the bloodstream.

When hormones are taken by mouth, they are processed through an entirely different pathway in the body—the digestive tract and then the liver.

- **Poor absorption.** Oral estrogen tablets may not be fully dissolved if a woman is taking antacids or has naturally low stomach acid. When that occurs, she won't be getting the full benefit of the estrogen.

- **Risk of blood clots.** Estrogen taken orally delivers a high dose of hormones directly to the liver. This changes the way the liver functions and in a small percentage of women alters the body's chemistry, resulting in a greater tendency to form blood clots in veins and arteries and cause heart attacks.

The Aging Factor

In spite of these concerns, until age 70, women taking equine estrogen had better health than those taking no hormones at all.

As women age, if they have been taking equine estrogen, it is advisable for them to stop taking oral hormones and switch to transdermal bioidenticals sometime between 60 and 70.

Older women over 60 taking oral equine estrogen have an increased risk for blood clots and stroke of about 2 in 100. Many women look at these numbers and don't worry a bit. Others look at the same numbers and stop taking their oral hormones right away and switch to transdermals. Absorbed through the skin, transdermals avoid harmful effects on the liver and do not have a clotting risk.

We are all unique in our values and the way in which we respond to these facts. A good provider's job is to inform you of your options, based on the vast amounts of data, and help you make sense of them. You are the decision-maker. Your opinion counts 100 percent.

Confusing Chemistry

One of the biggest issues with equine estrogen and synthetic progestin (MPA) is the fact that they differ from our own hormones in important ways.

Premarin

The composition of a mare's hormones is vastly different than that of a woman. They contain more than 400 different compounds not found in human estrogen. Whether or not this makes a big difference to your health has yet to be scientifically determined.

In a mare's body, the primary estrogen is estrone (E1), a minor player among human estrogens. In the human body, this creates estrone levels as high as 90 percent, quite different than our own normal balance of estrogens. The estrone must be converted in the liver to estradiol, a process involving several steps. Although women on Premarin do not typically develop liver problems, this does place an extra burden on the liver. Other mare's estrogens include equilin, which is foreign to the human body and may have effects different from our own estrogens.

Provera

Marketed as Provera, this progestin is a synthetic variation of the hormone progesterone. (The chemical name is medroxy progesterone acetate or MPA for short.) This little chemical is essential for the safe use of estrogen and does a great job in preventing uterine cancer.

Unfortunately, this hormone formula has a downside. When taken continuously on a daily basis, it raises the risk of heart disease. Risk factors include higher blood fats—such as harmful LDL cholesterol and triglycerides—as well as markers of inflammation. Due to these risks, progestin (MPA) is no longer considered the preferred form of progestin or progesterone.

The First Estrogens from Plants

The next development in estrogen products was the synthesis of conjugated estrogens derived from plants. These estrogens were based on the formula of Premarin, because it had been so successful in treating menopause symptoms. The plant-derived estrogens contain a mix of the same eight primary estrogens found in Premarin.

Plant-derived estrogens are not drawn from animal extracts, so they do not contain the hundreds of other compounds found in Premarin. These plant-based estrogens are used in the same dosage as Premarin and carry the same recommendations for prevention of uterine lining overgrowth. Progestin (MPA) is recommended for use in combination with the plant-based conjugates, on a cyclical or continuous schedule, which is essential for women with a uterus.

Hormone Tips

Your responses to hormones are unique to you and your chemistry, so a certain amount of trial and error is part of finding the right fit. A trial period of three months can be very helpful. Talk with your provider about the product most likely to be successful for you.

Advantages of All Estrogens

Equine estrogen offers many of the advantages found in all safe forms of estrogen. As mentioned, research published in 2009 has shown that all forms of estrogen lower the risk of Alzheimer's disease, Parkinson's, and other dementias. Estrogens also decrease the risk of heart disease. Used in combination with progesterone, estrogen also reduces uterine cancer risk by approximately 20 percent. Equally impressive are the reductions in colon cancer and diabetes. Most encouraging of all are estrogen's protective effects against osteoporosis. Current FDA guidelines for estrogens have confirmed the safety and effectiveness of these hormones for the prevention of bone loss.

Chapter 3

Why Bioidenticals May Be Better

In This Chapter

- What are bioidenticals and how do they compare with conventional HRT?
- How bioidenticals ease periomenopause
- How bioidenticals solve the riddle of full menopause
- Why women prefer bioidenticals for graceful aging

The past 70 years have been a time of incredible scientific innovation. Just think of a manual typewriter from 1942 compared to any laptop computer with WiFi. Contrast a rotary dial phone with your cell phone today. In terms of science, since the 1940s we've put a man on the moon, transplanted the human heart, and mapped the human genome. During this time researchers have also defined the structure of human hormones with absolute precision. As a result, we are now able to reproduce hormone molecules in their purest form.

The first commercial estrogen product was released almost 70 years ago. With the limited science of the time, this product was definitely a breakthrough. However, today we have a much greater understanding of the body's complex, elegant chemistry. The availability of products that precisely duplicate a woman's hormones enables us to provide hormone therapy without the side effects of earlier products.

What Are Bioidenticals?

The newest generation of hormone products is described as bioidenticals because their structure duplicates the composition of human hormones exactly, atom for atom. Bioidentical hormones have full FDA approval and are manufactured to the highest pharmaceutical standards, created from plant molecules. More than 800 research studies conducted worldwide have shown the safety of bioidenticals. The hormones reproduced in bioidentical formulas include three types of estrogen: estrone (E1), estradiol (E2), and estriol (E3), as well as progesterone and testosterone.

- **Bioidentical estradiol.** This form of estrogen is your most potent natural hormone. Your body converts estradiol into the other two major types of estrogen—estriol and estrone—so you have the complete mix of estrogens in your bloodstream. Bioidentical estradiol can be taken through a skin patch, cream, gel, spray, or vaginally using a ring or a tiny vaginal tablet.

- **Bioidentical progesterone.** This form of progesterone duplicates your own and has been shown to be much safer than synthetic progestin (MPA) because bioidenticals do not carry the risk of overworking your liver. In menopause we use bioidentical progesterone for its potentially lifesaving properties in preventing uterine cancer. There are rigorous standards for prescribing progesterone to counterbalance estradiol, so the dosage and schedule you and your doctor select must be adhered to carefully. Bioidentical progesterone is taken orally in tablet form or vaginally as a tablet or gel.

- **Bioidentical testosterone.** Many women are surprised to learn that our bodies produce a certain amount of testosterone. This is actually a key hormone for women as well as men—one that maintains muscle mass (keeping you strong and trim), supports your libido, and helps you stay mentally alert, at the top of your game. Bioidentical testosterone products supply the level of natural testosterone produced in a woman's body by her ovaries and adrenal glands.

Irene had a very late menopause. The "Energizer Bunny" of menstruation, at 59 she had her last period. Shocked when night sweats robbed her of her sleep, her interest in sex, and her self-confidence, she confided, "It was as though a veil had descended on me." Six weeks after starting a low dose of daily estradiol gel, (simply applied to her thigh), she was back to normal. A little estradiol can make a big difference.

It's fascinating to think that a product with such practical human applications is the result of so much careful scientific research. Bioidenticals were first developed in pharmacological laboratories and are produced in highly specialized industrial facilities. Plant extracts, primarily yam and soy, provide the molecules that are converted into exact replicas of our naturally occurring hormones. The bioidentical manufacturers that produce FDA-approved products adhere to the highest standards for consumer protection. These hormones then go through a series of state-of-the-art tests to verify chemical stability, batch-to-batch uniformity, and overall product quality.

Hormone Tips

Specialized delivery systems are used to provide timed-release products taken orally, transdermally, or vaginally. Estradiol patches have this slow-release technology built in, so the hormone can be gradually absorbed through the skin. In oral products, the micronization protects the hormone against stomach acid. Progesterone tablets (used orally or vaginally) are micronized by coating the individual hormone molecules with oil (typically peanut, canola, or sesame) to support gradual, even absorption. The vaginal tablets are concentrated in a slow-release product the size of a baby aspirin.

In the development of bioidenticals, these delivery systems were one of the big hurdles researchers had to overcome. It took years of rigorous science to develop all the mechanisms involved in each complex product, particularly those with timed release.

Bioidenticals or Conventional HRT?

Bioidenticals are easier to explain than the equine estrogen in Premarin because bioidentical estradiol is identical to the estradiol in your own body. In contrast, when you use Premarin, you're consuming more than 400 chemicals that are not native to your body and that you don't really need. Bioidentical hormones are designed to match your chemistry exactly, with none of the side effects.

Steady as You Go

Your body loves continuity. Although you can accommodate changes in hormone levels, your body loves the feeling of being consistent, because you function best when your hormones are within a certain range, "in the groove." (We've all had those days when we feel tranquil and everything seems effortless.) After you've achieved your ideal balance, you can get on with your life.

You want to stay on that sweet spot, with hormone levels that are constant and stable over the course of the day. Using a bioidentical with a timed-release gives you that continuity. An estradiol patch, for example, provides slow, continuous release through your skin, avoiding the unnatural peaks and valleys of estrogen that would occur if you were taking it by mouth, once or twice a day.

Before menopause, your hormone levels changed at different times during the month, but they did not bounce up and down from hour to hour. Pills or tablets that you take by mouth cause a see-saw of estrogen levels over the course of a day. For some women this is not a problem, but for others it can result in mood swings, crankiness, erratic sleep, or occasional hot flashes.

Better Balance

Bioidenticals also support a good balance of other hormones such as thyroid (an important hormone that's not tied to reproduction). This is really appreciated by women on thyroid supplements, because their levels are adjusted and monitored very carefully. In contrast, Premarin, taken orally, can bind up "free" thyroid and sex hormones, essentially taking them out of action. Free levels of testosterone are also important, not just for libido, but also for good muscle tone and weight control.

When a hormone is bound, it's like catching a baseball and then holding on to it and not releasing it back into the game. Imagine your hormones as little baseballs. Some are in the catcher's mitt, ready to be released when you need them (these are the "bound" hormones). Others are in play on the field, creating the effects of an energetic day (these are your "free" hormones). We need hormones available in both states. The balance between the reservoir of inactive "bound" hormones and the available active "free" hormones can be a delicate dance for some women.

Jaime at 51 had the "full Monty of menopause," as she put it. "My joints ache, my hair is falling out, I can't sleep. I can't even wear my contact lenses, because my eyes are so dry. Oh yes, and my husband wanted me to ask about sex, because that's gone out the window too." Thinking over the best approach for Jaime, I knew that she'd been on thyroid replacement for 16 years since her last child was born. Getting her thyroid right had been tricky for her internist, because she had an auto-immune condition. To avoid any changes in her thyroid balance, I recommended bioidentical estradiol taken through the skin (she chose a patch that just gets changed twice a week) plus cyclic monthly progesterone. That was all she needed, since her own testosterone level was still fine. When I saw her in six weeks, she was "back to good." She'd already begun shedding some of that perimenopause weight and confided, "My marriage is the best it's been in years!"

Quality and Constancy

Bioidentical hormones are guaranteed to be exactly identical every time. The FDA requires this oversight through multi-step laboratory testing during manufacturing. On the other hand, hormones derived from animals in products such as Premarin can have variations due to seasonal changes and the metabolism of the individual animal. Thus there may be product variations or lot batch differences. Bioidenticals are absolutely consistent every time.

Thriving in Perimenopause

Sleepless nights, hot flashes, night sweats, and mood swings … your days are hard enough without these hassles and aggravations. Bioidenticals make it possible for you to function again.

Bioidenticals are just the thing to smooth out the early symptoms of menopause when a woman's cycle first becomes irregular or erratic. Just a little bioidentical estradiol can resolve the insomnia and night sweats triggered before a menstrual period.

Long before a woman's final period, her hormones can become amazingly unpredictable. (This may even start 10 years before actual full-blown menopause. The final period comes at the end of the process, not at the beginning.) Some women find their lives fraught with anxiety and tumult, because their hormone levels are all over the map. In our 20s and 30s, our hormone levels gracefully rise during the course of a month from a high of 500 during ovulation to a low of about 30 or 40pg/dl right before a period. The effects of this low are reflected in the symptoms of PMS. In perimenopause, these levels may spike into the thousands, with totally unnerving effects. This creates mood swings that resemble PMS on steroids. Sometimes breasts are busting out of your bra, and you may feel so bloated that you wonder if you're pregnant. Yet with the onset of menopause, these same hormones may crash as low as 10 or 15 pg/dl.

Unfortunately, there's no flashing red light that tells us, "Hey, Honey! Your hormones are whacked!"

With bioidenticals, we can now smooth out these ups and downs by supporting your cycle with a healthy level of estradiol that allows you to sleep again, so you can navigate the storms of perimenopause without feeling so jostled.

Bioidenticals in forms such as patch, gel, or spray provide solutions that are safe and effective, with positive resonance in all the areas of a woman's life. The less we notice our hormones, the better we feel. In fact, throughout our lives it is only when something is not working that we even notice it. Praise our natural hormones that they worked so well and so effortlessly for so long! But when we head into menopause, all bets are off. The "Pause" can trigger rollercoaster moods, anxiety, and other unpleasant symptoms. Low-dose bioidentical therapy is often very useful in taming these moods.

Hormone Tips

Many women need low-dose birth control hormones to adequately treat the wild swings of perimenopause, especially those who have extremely heavy bleeding. Interestingly, as women approach age 50, many report hot flashes and night sweats, even while they're on active contraceptive hormones. A little bioidentical estradiol, used continuously, can help women with this experience stay asleep and avoid hot flashes.

Mastering Full Menopause

Finessing the territory of menopause requires new skills. In younger years we never had to think about taking a hormone simply to get a good night of sleep or keeping the vagina moist and bladder comfy. For many it comes as a rude shock to be so dependent on a prescription. Many women report that this is the first "drug," they've ever taken on a regular basis other than contraceptives.

Smoother Moods

Your moods are often intimately linked to your hormone balance. Because estradiol is the ultimate secret to tranquility, it's not surprising that many women on bioidenticals experience more tranquil moods. Transdermals offer smooth, reliable delivery of estradiol, making it available to every cell in your body and brain.

In comparison, hormones taken orally can bounce moods around. For some women the formula of Premarin seems to cause negative emotional shifts, even when it takes care of hot flashes and sleep problems. In addition, the progestin (MPA) in PremPro is well known to trigger depression in some women. Be aware that if a woman forgets to take her daily pill, blood level variations can cause emotional symptoms such as crying jags and the blues. (Transdermal patches are a good solution to the human failing of forgetting meds, which is most likely to happen when one has the blahs.) If your mood "could be better," bioidenticals may be worth trying.

Better Libido and Sex

When it comes to sex, bioidentical estrogen is often prescribed with testosterone to support a healthy libido. Production of testosterone by your ovaries falls steadily in menopause. That's why most of us need to add back what was lost. The adrenals make a little testosterone, but not enough for optimal balance after 50. Supplementing testosterone has been shown to enhance satisfaction in sex better than herbs, vitamins, or a placebo, especially in women with testosterone blood levels at the lowest third of normal range. Bioidentical testosterone is prescribed in a definable dosage that can be adjusted as needed, so you get enough, but not too much. With bioidentical testosterone, it sometimes takes several weeks of trial and error to get the dosage exactly right. Approved doses of testosterone aim to achieve predictable testosterone levels that duplicate those found in healthy women.

The equine hormones in Premarin include a certain amount of testosterone-like hormone, because horses have their own natural androgens (hormones that have similar effects to those of testosterone). Some of these androgens get excreted in their urine. However, Premarin does not contain a pure form of testosterone that is measurable or predictable.

In addition, Premarin has a tendency to bind hormones, which can actually drop the level of free testosterone in the body, making it less available to support good health or good sex. As a result, libido and responsiveness may become lackluster in women with low or borderline testosterone (that means most women after menopause). When too much testosterone is bound, not enough circulates freely in the brain or body to support satisfying sex. Most women need a minimum of free and active testosterone to sparkle and maintain a playful interest in sex.

Warning Label

Free levels of testosterone are important, not just for libido, but also for good bone density, muscle tone, and weight control. Binding up your testosterone can cause everything from insomnia to lack of assertiveness. In contrast to the androgens in conventional hormones, bioidenticals deliver testosterone through timed-release and gradual absorption, so they don't interfere with other complex processes going on throughout the body.

The testosterone that American men have used in patches for the past 30 years is all bioidentical but in doses that are 10 times too strong for women. (So don't borrow your husband's T-patch or you may get some hairy side effects you didn't really want!)

Smart and Safe

Given the benefits of bioidenticals, it's worth taking a little time to "get it right." Initially, there may be a brief period of adjustment. Hormone receptors can change when a woman has been without normal levels of circulating estradiol and progesterone for a long time. When she re-starts, she may feel slightly out of balance in subtle ways for a period of a few weeks or for several weeks.

This can almost always be avoided by starting at the very lowest dose. This enables you to raise your hormone levels gradually and can support a surprising level of comfort from the very beginning.

Your body chemistry is as unique as your fingerprints, so the goal is to achieve the right balance for *you*. Some women find that the mixture of estrogens in conventional hormones is a better match for their metabolism. For the vast majority of women, bioidenticals feel just like their own chemistry and provide a sweet sense of inner balance and well-being that extends through full menopause and beyond.

Less Breast Cancer

To our enormous relief, studies during the past decade report about 20 percent lower incidence of breast cancer in women who have used bioidentical estradiol and bioidentical progesterone for more than five years. In contrast, PremPro, which is equine estrogen with progestin (MPA), negated the lower rate of breast cancer.

When it comes to breast cancer, there are two important points to think about. First, the original findings from the study that reported the breast cancer story were totally reversed when the researchers reanalyzed the data. Yet when have you *ever* seen a headline that announced, "No Cancer Risk!"? The second point is that all the studies that suggested a link between estrogen and cancer were conducted with oral Premarin and PremPro. The studies used estrogen from horse's urine, which has a chemical make-up that is incredibly different than a woman's own estrogens. Premarin and PremPro are both given by mouth, which clearly has effects on liver function. None of the negative breast cancer findings that have caused so much alarm were conducted with bioidenticals. Clinical trials using bioidenticals are consistently reassuring in their positive outcomes and reports of decreased risk.

In Debbie's case, it had been seven years since she was cured of a tiny spot of DCIS (ductal carcinoma in situ), the most common early pre-cancer found by mammograms. She was only 46 then and still having regular periods. Now 53 and fully menopausal, she described disabling hot flashes by day and drenching sweats by night. "Honestly, the lumpectomy was nothing compared to the energy drain and brain fog I've been going through." We discussed her options, especially in light of the very clear scientific data that women with previous diagnoses of DCIS are fine candidates for bioidentical estrogen. "Yes, I realize that, because I already consulted with the cancer risk genetic counselor who told me the same thing. In fact she gave me your name and mentioned that you helped establish a comprehensive breast health center. She said you would know what is safe." Debbie began using an estradiol spray, and got some relief, but wanted a higher dose to get rid of hot flashes completely and restore vaginal moisture. The vaginal ring, Femring, was perfect because she traveled a great deal with a busy job and only needed to change it every three months. She cycled with bioidentical progesterone monthly and life was good again.

Aging Gracefully

The ideal hormone supplement addresses your symptoms and protects your health without adverse effects. The safe use of bioidentical estradiol and progesterone at every age has been shown to protect women against many of the disorders of aging, from Alzheimer's disease and Parkinson's to osteoporosis and hip fractures. Bioidentical estradiol also offers protective effects against several types of cancer, including uterine, colon, and invasive breast cancer. Bioidenticals, absorbed through the skin, do not increase the tendency to form blood clots, in contrast to hormones taken orally, such as Premarin.

Healthy Hearts

If your family history includes heart disease, you could have an increased genetic risk for cardiovascular disease. In that case, you may be one of the patients who opts for hormone replacement as a form of prevention, even if you currently have very few symptoms. A growing body of convincing data confirms this protective effect.

Heart health benefits of bioidenticals include improved levels of good cholesterol (HDL), less harmful cholesterol (LDL), and lower risk of heart disease.

In contrast, PremPro (not a bioidentical) has been found to have increased risks due to the progestin content (MPA). These unwanted effects include elevated harmful triglycerides and cholesterol (LDL), and markers of inflammation, reflected in higher C-reactive protein levels. The PEPI trial, published in 1995, showed important differences in heart disease risk according to the type of progestin used in combination with estrogen.

The Esther research study, published in 2007, confirmed that women using transdermal bioidentical estradiol had fewer blood clots compared to those taking equine estrogens. More good news from the same research group is that the use of bioidentical progesterone does not change this highly positive data. In contrast, taking Premarin by mouth increases clotting risk sixfold, 10 times that seen with bioidentical estradiol taken orally.

Brain Power

Bioidenticals have a greater protective effect against strokes caused by blood clots than oral conjugated estrogens. Because blood pressure tends to be safely lowered in women on bioidentical estradiol, there is also less risk of hemorrhagic strokes. In addition, the protective effects against weight gain further reduce these risks.

Women on bioidenticals in large research trials do not have the tendency to deep vein thrombosis, which involves blood clots in the large veins and other clot-related health problems. Many women look at the bluish "varicose veins" they can see on their legs and are relieved to learn that they do not cause medical problems. However, what would be a source of concern is any type of clotting that might occur in the deeper veins in the legs, pelvis, or even the brain. These clots are often tremendously painful, so they do not go unnoticed.

Monique came to see me after six weeks of agonizing night sweats, feeling "hotter than July. My husband says he's fine, still sleeping cozy under the down comforter, but I wake up at 2:30 A.M. wondering if I am coming down with the flu." I knew that her mom at 70 had been diagnosed with Parkinson's disease, so Monique and her daughter had gotten genetic testing. Her test results showed a gene that indicates a high risk for blood clots. As a result, Monique is not a candidate for Premarin because it increases the risk for a blood clot. Our choice was clear: bioidentical estradiol using a skin patch to give her quick relief from the "raging fires of night sweats" and restore her sleep, without increasing her risk for clots or phlebitis. We balanced that prescription with bioidentical progesterone taken every month. Within a few weeks she was sleeping through the night, "cool as a cucumber, happy as a clam."

Why Women Prefer Bioidenticals

Bioidenticals are exact replicas of our own hormones, tested by natural biologic processes for millions of years. It makes sense to replace hormones in the same form as those in the body, to re-create your own "natural" estrogen state.

A transitional three months of "trying it on for size" can be helpful. You'll want to have an open discussion with your provider about the product most likely to be successful for you. About 95 percent of the women who opt for bioidenticals find that they are a good match. That's a batting average of 950! Any baseball player would love to have that rate of home runs!

Today you have a range of choices. Sixty years ago, Premarin and Provera were the only options available, so women had no way to compare their effects with other approaches to hormone therapy. Now, if one formula doesn't fit your body's chemistry, you can ask your provider to prescribe another. All the FDA-approved hormones today are very safe for the average woman entering menopause. Ultimately, you want to work with your provider and monitor your own unique response. Honoring your personal needs is at the heart of good self-care.

Right Provider, Right Product

In This Chapter

- The importance of being seen in person by a health professional
- Suggestions on what to look for in a provider, especially if you'd like to use bioidenticals
- The most important reasons to think twice before using a mail-order pharmacy for your prescription
- A checklist you can use to help you select safe, effective products

Consumers and physicians are often surprised to learn that bioidentical hormones are manufactured by leading pharmaceutical companies, available by prescription from their neighborhood pharmacy. In some cases, consumers don't realize that their trusted hormone patch is actually a bioidentical product. Others may not realize that the estrogen cream they are using to improve their sex life could also be protecting them against Alzheimer's disease and osteoporosis.

Bioidentical formulas are among the safest hormone products ever developed. However, despite an exceptional 20-year record of safety, bioidenticals are sometimes used in the wrong way, or under the wrong circumstances. When that happens, it puts a woman's health at risk. Every week, I see patients who have health issues because they weren't using the right hormone products. Often this is because some physicians, nurse practitioners, osteopaths, and complementary providers are not yet fully informed about the data and the safest protocols for hormone use.

One of the issues involves patients who purchase hormone products based on a phone consultation with a provider who has never seen them. Another involves hormones prescribed by a physician who knows the patient, but not the new products. The third issue involves products purchased from mail-order and Internet compounding pharmacies.

A heart-breaking example of this problem is a woman I saw recently who had developed uterine cancer. Her bioidentical sublingual drops did not include the progesterone it claimed to contain. In addition to this error, she had not had a pelvic exam in seven years, which would have picked up her cancer at a much earlier stage.

If you're interested in taking bioidenticals, you can obtain a list of certified menopause practitioners who are highly knowledgeable about the use of these hormones. The most comprehensive list currently available to the public can be obtained through the North American Menopause Society, www.menopause.org. Websites that focus on consumer safety and not selling a product are the most reliable sources of information. Beware web marketing, as it is deliberately designed to get your business, not necessarily support optimal safety.

Personal Care vs. Phone Consult

If you're considering using hormones, you really need to be seen in person before you do. That means a local physician or provider, rather than a doctor who provides care at a distance by phone or e-mail. If you use a physician who writes you a prescription without ever seeing you, that person will not know your health history or your family risk factors. If they have not examined you, they may not be aware of important physical findings and symptoms. All these potential risk factors need to be taken into consideration before writing a prescription.

When a woman obtains a prescription through a phone consult with a doctor who has never examined her, important steps are neglected:

- There is no way to verify the credentials or expertise of the provider.
- A pelvic exam will not be provided.
- The practitioner will not know the patient's medical history in depth.

- The provider will not have access to her records or the results from her blood tests.
- There will be no in-person follow-up to monitor her safety.

A face-to-face office visit gives the provider a level of understanding that's just not possible on the phone. Sarah's case demonstrates this clearly. In a recent office visit, she requested a hormone prescription hoping that it would resolve her insomnia. As part of her gynecological checkup, a careful breast exam revealed a tiny thickening—smaller than the size of a pea. It turned out to be very early breast cancer that hadn't shown up on her mammogram 10 months earlier. The lump was easily and successfully removed in come-and-go surgery and she is enjoying disease-free life seven years later. That is the value of actually being seen by the provider who prescribes your hormones.

Finding the Right Provider

The first step in getting the right prescription is to work with the right provider. You need a health professional who has the legal capacity to write prescriptions. This means a medical doctor (M.D.), a doctor of osteopathy (D.O.), or a nurse practitioner who can write prescriptions under the supervision of an M.D. or a D.O. Chiropractors do not have the legal scope of practice to write prescriptions. You also want the safest, most effective hormone products available, so you don't want to get side-tracked by experimenting with a whole variety of over-the-counter herbs that are not likely to work.

Optimal health care is based on a genuine partnership with your doctor or practitioner. You want a provider who knows the research. If you're going to use bioidenticals, you need someone who is current on hormone prescribing in general and bioidenticals in particular. Also bear in mind that a physician in another state cannot order blood tests to check your hormone levels, do follow-ups, breast exams, sonograms, or biopsies to check the health of your uterine lining.

Getting rid of symptoms is easy. The challenge is to get a prescription that relieves your symptoms, safeguards your health, and is tailored to your needs. Sometimes this is a tall order.

The Provider's Credentials

You'll want to keep a few standards in mind when selecting a provider. Do they have training from an accredited institution? Do they hold a professional license in good standing? What are their credentials in terms of hormone therapy? If you have a serious problem, how would this provider resolve it? Are they well networked with specialists?

Are they board-certified by one of the professional organizations that evaluates specialists in the fields of medicine through the American Board of Medical Specialists? Accredited endocrinologists and gynecologists both have this special designation. Board certification affirms the expertise of the physician, which is an added protection for consumers. Often you can learn this type of information from a provider's website or their brochure. Many physicians' offices have a patient coordinator or new-patient representative who will take the time to answer this type of question for you.

Have they had recent professional training to stay current with the research and protocol for hormones? Has the provider attended a course held by a professional society such as the American College of OB/GYN or the North American Menopause Society?

On the other hand, do they simply hold a certificate from a weekend course such as those offered by mail-order compounding pharmacies? There are big financial incentives and profit motives that encourage less-skilled providers to "get on the bandwagon," writing prescriptions for bioidentical hormones. Buyer beware.

Knowledge of Bioidenticals

This is a rapidly changing field. Many family doctors, general practitioners, internists, and gynecologists are becoming well informed and know the fine points of prescribing hormones. But others don't.

Often problems begin with a prescription by a practitioner who knows the field in general. They may know *you* well, but may not be up on the research and new product data. If their prescription does not include the right form of progesterone, in the right amount, that will put you at risk. If you have any questions or concerns about your prescription, now or later, be sure to get a second opinion rather than take a chance.

When you're actually meeting with the provider, notice whether they can discuss the benefits and downside of various products. That is often a sign that they track the research (although not always). They know which products are appropriate, and for which patients. Of course, you won't know this until you're actually sitting in their office. To be sure you have someone knowledgeable, check the list from the North American Menopause Society, or get a referral from a physician you respect.

Getting a Physical

You want to be sure that the prescriber knows your health history and that of your closest family. If you see them in person, they can order comprehensive lab work and discuss the results with you. Ideally your provider is someone who will pay careful attention to any medical problems that might come up and also address your concerns. Every medical encounter is a chance to prevent disease. Ideally your bioidentical doc will communicate with your primary care physician to be sure your total health is addressed and enhanced.

Getting the Right Prescription

You want the right product for *you*, given your health history. For example, if you are still perimenopausal, (less than a year since your last menstrual period) bioidentical hormones may not control irregular cycles or abnormal bleeding. On the other hand, although they will not control your cycle, they are often very effective in decreasing other symptoms.

Writing a prescription for bioidenticals always involves more than just filling a prescription. When I saw Jean for the first time, she just wanted an old prescription refilled. She was using bioidentical estrogen capsules (taken by mouth). Yet her new patient questionnaire showed a strong family history of stroke and phlebitis. Her blood test showed that she had inherited a high risk for clotting. So giving her hormones by mouth (either Premarin *or* bioidenticals) would have put her at even higher risk for a life-threatening problem. The best prescription for a woman in this situation is a transdermal patch, gel, or transvaginal product. Jean was spared a potentially devastating illness simply by changing her hormone prescription. Six years later, she's alive and well.

Hormone Tips

More is not necessarily better. For example, you want to avoid too much testosterone, because it can cause thinning of the hair on your head, excessive hair growth in other places where you don't want it, or a bad complexion. You also want to avoid too much progesterone, because that can make your hair fall out or cause depression. Yet the prescription needs to be strong enough to address your symptoms and protect you long-term.

At the end of the day, you want to know that you're taking the right hormone, in the right form, at the right dosage.

Ongoing Follow-Ups

It's important that you be seen for follow-up within one to three months, just to assure that the new plan is working. You may have other issues or symptoms that need to be monitored (including conditions with no symptoms at all). For example, was there a yeast infection or irritation? You want to make sure that the symptoms and physical findings discussed in the initial exam are resolved.

Some issues just aren't picked up in a phone consult. A woman may feel fine, even when there's a smoldering problem. In Tiffany's case, it became clear on her first visit that she was having a great deal of abnormal bleeding, which she thought was her "period." A sonogram confirmed that her uterine lining had grown dangerously thick, putting her at risk of cancer. Although the biopsy showed extensive overgrowth, fortunately there was no cancer. With the appropriate hormone prescription, her uterine lining gradually returned to normal, and she continues to be healthy four years later.

If you are interested in taking bioidenticals, you want to be sure that you're getting the right prescription. The following checklist will help ensure that this happens:

1. Is your doctor knowledgeable about bioidenticals? Sometimes docs want to make

you happy but really don't know a lot about the hormones a patient asks for. If you find you're being seen by a provider who really isn't knowledgeable, it's okay to work with them short-term, but be sure to get a referral to a doctor that specializes in women's health care.

2. Can your provider offer comprehensive care for all problems that may arise as a result of prescribing this hormone? They need to understand your hormone chemistry, track your liver function, know how to interpret various blood tests, and interpret an ultrasound image.

3. Will you be getting a follow-up exam and periodic check-ups to keep an eye on your health? Be sure that routine health screenings are also part of your health care. For a comprehensive list of screenings, see www. DrRicki.com.

4. If your prescription is a compounded cream, is it from a local pharmacy you and your personal physician know and trust? What information indicates that this cream has better effectiveness or is safer than those that have passed FDA scrutiny? In the case of testosterone cream, there is no FDA product currently available that is specifically for women.

5. If you have never had a hysterectomy, is adequate progesterone included in the prescription, either cyclically or continuously?

You never want to hear, "Oops, I forgot to prescribe your progesterone and that is why you are bleeding."

6. Does your prescription have the right dosage of estrogen to take care of your symptoms, without elevating these levels too high? The FDA's recommendation is "The lowest effective dose for the period of time required to meet treatment goals."

Mail-Order Pharmacies

Currently, mail-order pharmacies are one of the primary sources of bioidentical products, in part because women (and sometimes their doctors) don't realize they can get excellent bioidenticals through their neighborhood drug store.

There are several issues that relate to the use of a mail-order pharmacy. The first, which we've described, is the lack of patient monitoring. The other is the question of unsupervised prescription products.

Almost every week a new patient comes to me who has been using a compounded preparation, and has hormone levels that are far too high or too low. Many of these patients have been using products purchased by phone or on the Internet. If the actual product does not match the prescription, hormone levels may really miss the mark. If a disease results years later, where will the mail-order company be?

Warning Label

Sometimes a simple hormone cream can become a matter of life and death. Compounded hormone creams are not always reliable—especially those obtained with a provider who has never seen you, from a mail-away pharmacy. There may not be enough progesterone in the cream to protect you effectively—or it may not be in a usable bioactive form. Taking an inappropriate product or prescription—year in, year out—can put you at real risk.

The original intent of compounding pharmacy laws was to provide a facility where pharmacists could make preparations to meet uncommon but specific patient needs. Traditionally, this is done under a doctor's close supervision, by a highly knowledgeable compounding pharmacist. For decades, these pharmacists, working in concert with gynecologists and other care providers, have been developing highly customized prescriptions to meet patients' unique individual needs, without raising concerns by the FDA. It is the close and authentic medical supervision by the treating physician that makes these compounding pharmacy-patient-physician relationships work for each woman's best outcome.

The issues with *mail-order* compounding pharmacies are that they may not have adequate supervision, and because they are providing services at a distance, there is limited accountability. Those that market on the Internet also make unsubstantiated health claims.

Mail-order compounding pharmacies frequently promote direct-to-consumer marketing of prescription hormone products. They take an approach comparable to multi-level marketing, which has traditionally been used for over-the-counter products such as vitamins, cosmetics, and household cleaning products. In the case of bioidenticals, what is being aggressively marketed is prescription medication.

Another key issue here is the prescribing of bio-identicals incorrectly without direct patient care or follow-up. Estrogen taken alone without progesterone relieves symptoms, so initially these women do well and are satisfied customers. However, long-term use of estrogen without progesterone causes a silent build-up of the uterine lining, without any awareness on the part of the patient. (Many women, but not all, will bleed or spot, a warning sign that there is a potential problem. Those who do not have symptoms will have no awareness that they are developing cancer.)

This incorrect prescribing has resulted in tragic increases in uterine cancer. These questionable practices have placed the agressive mail-order compounding pharmacies under greater scrutiny, which is ultimately for your protection as a consumer.

Safe, Effective Products

Safety must be documented for any product you use long-term. This means that the product is made in a totally reliable, verifiable manner, with complete purity. You want a product that provides a consistent dosage with predictable absorption and distribution in your body. One of the keys to product safety is confidence in the manufacturer, the integrity of their products, and the reliability of their quality assurance. Bioidentical hormones that are FDA-approved hold a guarantee of purity and absolute consistency, batch after batch.

FDA-Approved Hormone Products

Overall, *FDA approval* works for your benefit, even if the pace is frustratingly slow now and then. This approval process gives consumers assurance that what is in this bottle, pill, cream, gel, ring, or patch has effects in your body that are safe and predictable. Stories of tainted prescription medications exported from China remind us of the importance of FDA controls. Thousands of women and years of research go into every FDA-approved hormone product before it becomes available as a prescription product in your local pharmacy.

def•i•ni•tion

> There are four major steps in **FDA ap-proval:** Phase 1 involves testing a new medication in human subjects to determine safety and tolerability. Phase 2 research focuses on whether the drug actually works, and defines the effective dose. Phase 3 is a clinical study conducted in a hospital or outpatient setting; and Phase 4 involves ongoing review and monitoring. Today this process costs approximately $50 million and is required in order to bring a new drug to market.

Can It Be Traced?

Reliable medications are completely traceable from start to finish. That means that you, the patient, can look at a product label and find its lot number and expiration date. The same is true for pills or capsules. Even tiny individual pills have a code printed on them so you can verify what they are. (*The Physician's Desk Reference* has thousands of pictures of individual prescription items, as does the Internet.) This makes it possible, 100 percent of the time, to trace any product to a particular manufacturer, location, date, and product batch. You need this level of accountability, especially if you are going to use a product or medication long-term. It is cause for concern when there is no label, identifying lot number, expiration date, source code, or product insert.

Take the time you need to find the right health-care solutions for these issues. Like most midlife women, you probably keep a busy pace. Don't discard safety for quick fixes. A commitment to quality care now is your best insurance for better health in the "golden girl" years ahead. If you've devoted yourself to solving life's problems, this is your chance to savor a new sense of freedom and enjoy the sweet moments life has to offer. Make it a point to write yourself into the schedule each day. Self-care is primary care.

Chapter 5

Your Personal Plan

In This Chapter

- When to supplement estrogen
- How to work with your care provider
- What information you'll need for an office visit
- How to track your symptoms
- Which lab tests may be ordered
- What factors are key in selecting safe, effective hormone products

Women love having choices. From the color of our hair to the furnishings that we choose to decorate our homes, it's all about choices. When it comes to hormones, we also want a range of choices to meet our own unique needs.

This chapter walks you through some of the choices involved in your hormone decisions, with an emphasis on bioidentical choices. The goal is to provide you with both insight and the nitty-gritty details you need to be an active partner in your health care. This will enable you to work with your provider in developing a personalized health plan with wisdom and confidence.

When to Start?

Some aspects of health and hormone planning are the same for all women, but other elements will be somewhat unique to you. Think of menopause in terms of *your* own specific goals for your life. One of the factors to think about first is your age.

Your 40s: Perimenopause

If you're in your 40s, you'll want to educate yourself about perimenopause. You want to know the signs of this transition into menopause and their importance in terms of your health.

The medical literature is in complete agreement that timing is everything when it comes to hormone therapy and optimal health. The research has found that after a woman's hormone levels start dropping, the earlier she begins supplementing those hormones, the healthier she will remain. Ideally, even before you've gone six months or a year without a period, you'll want to see your doctor and address the ups and downs of falling estrogen levels as early as possible. In this initial phase, a very low dosage of estrogen support can make a major difference— smooth out the bumps in the road. Research shows that the earlier this support is started, the better women's health outcomes are both short- and long-term.

Your 50s: The Pause

The importance of starting early was the lesson learned in the largest study ever conducted on hormone therapy, which tracked the health of thousands of women for five years (the Women's Health Initiative, WHI). The younger women in the study derived the greatest benefits. Those who began hormone therapy within the first 10 years of menopause had the lowest rates of the diseases of aging. If you're still in your 50s, the research shows that your long-term health is better protected by supplementing your hormones than by avoiding hormone replacement. Even if you've gotten over the worst menopause symptoms such as hot flashes, you're likely to find that hormone therapy helps with weight control, increases energy, and improves your skin. We've already talked about the long-term health benefits. (See Chapters 1 through 3 for recaps.)

Your 60s: Start Low, Go Slow

For women who have taken a long break from hormone use, I advise starting with a very low dose of estrogen. Bioidentical estradiol can be taken through the skin, increasing the level gradually over time. Estrogen receptors change after many years when there is little or no estrogen in the body, so it's best to edge in gently, as we re-introduce these fundamental molecules.

How much is enough? Before menopause, our levels during our menstrual period were typically 30 to

40 pgm/ml (with a high of about 500 during ovulation). After menopause, many women average less than 10. The goal of hormone therapy is to relieve symptoms, usually achieved with estradiol blood levels of about 30 to 40 (estradiol is a woman's primary and most potent form of estrogen). "Start low and go slow" works best, increasing estradiol gradually until the symptoms are resolved. After you've achieved the appropriate level, you can switch to a tiny patch that you change twice a week, until you are at a dosage that meets the goal you and your provider have set. We don't need a blood test to tell us our symptoms are gone! Each one of us knows that for ourselves.

Your 70s: Ask Your Doctor

Women older than age 70 today may have been on and off estrogen for symptoms during their early years of menopause (usually Premarin or a related product). The consensus is that if you have been on estrogen and feel great, it's acceptable to continue taking it, but transition to a low-dose transdermal estradiol to keep risks as low as possible. For women who have not been on any type of estrogen product for more than 10 years, oral estrogen products are not advised. In terms of systemic use of transdermal estrogen, individual treatment decisions may vary and should be determined while working closely with a health-care provider. Estrogen use for older women is clearly the most appropriate when it addresses urinary symptoms or vaginal dryness, using locally applied or topical estrogen. Older women who need some vaginal estrogen treatment have a wide range of health-supporting choices, which are discussed in the product section, Using Bioidentical Hormones, that follows.

Working with Your Provider

You want a provider who is easy to work with. The best clinicians are open-minded, respectful of your ideas, and have the ability to communicate both information and life experience. You'll know when you're in the presence of a good listener and someone who's compassionate. You want someone who will consider every aspect of your life and your health—your life path as well as your health history and the health of your family. You want a flexible problem-solver who realizes that there is more than one way to do things.

Preparing for the Visit

You'll want to organize yourself and your information in advance of the office visit. This will help you get clearer on your goals and be better prepared. Physicians love well-organized patients, and your efforts will also help you get the most out of the visit.

- Be sure to order copies of your records well in advance and bring them with you.
- Make a separate list of all medications and supplements you're taking.
- Jot down your greatest concerns and put them in order of priority.

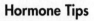

Hormone Tips

It helps to keep a chart or some type of diary of your symptoms. You can use a daily log, keep notes on the computer, or enter them in your Blackberry. Other useful approaches include a graph, a journal, a Daytimer, or a little calendar, such as the one found on DrRicki.com. The goal is to see if patterns emerge that you and your provider can address and resolve.

- Track your symptoms and health issues over time, in advance of your appointment.

- In terms of your health history, your provider needs to know if you have a history of thickening of the uterine lining, ovarian cysts, or a diagnosis of endometriosis. Endometriosis presents some particular considerations in menopause and in prescribing hormones. It's important to mention any surgeries, breast lumps, or abnormal pap smears

- It's important that your provider know whether either of your parents had heart disease, stroke, or gallbladder disease. Your clinician will also want to learn whether any of your close relatives have had cancer. Women who carry the genes for breast cancer and who used estrogen in menopause were found to have 50 percent *less* breast cancer.

A more proactive approach means that you are a true partner in your own health care. This is an opportunity to address the challenges of menopause and create a plan for resolving them. By gathering the information your provider needs to help you, you're setting the stage for the best possible outcome.

The Office Visit

You'll want to have a full gynecologic exam, which typically includes an annual pap smear. The person following your hormone prescription needs to have the skills to monitor the uterine lining, especially if abnormal bleeding occurs. When the uterine lining needs to be checked, a sample of the lining tissue (endometrial biopsy) can simply be taken in a miniaturized office procedure that can be done under local anesthesia quite comfortably in skilled hands. In most communities, this has replaced the vast majority of hospital-based D & Cs (dilation and curettage) that were once the primary way of making this assessment. Sonograms are also used to evaluate the status of the uterine lining.

The office visit is another opportunity to check your hormone prescriptions and see if they are meeting your needs. A breast exam should be included, at least once or optimally twice a year, as a gold standard. Mammograms are scheduled annually as they have been shown to lower the death rate from breast cancer. In the United States, happily, we have seen a steady decline in breast cancer death rates during the past 10 years, largely due to early detection because of mammograms.

Lab Tests: Pros and Cons

Most clinicians do not advise hormone testing. In fact, the most practical, cost-effective approach is simply a three-month trial with a hormone prescription. As surprising as this may seem, this is the standard of care. Sadly, there is no test on the market today that will fully predict your response to a specific hormone product. In some situations, doctors have been accused of padding their profits by ordering unnecessary lab tests.

Which Hormones?

Hormones, by definition, have an impact felt throughout the body. Your choice of hormones will influence all aspects of your health. These choices will also affect everything from your moods and your confidence to your total enjoyment of life. Even more importantly, hormones support optimal physical health and well-being.

Hormones by Mouth or Skin?

American women historically have preferred to take their hormones by mouth. This is changing. Research has shown clearly that some of the small but measurable risks of hormone replacement are lower when women take their hormones through the skin or vagina. Absorption through the skin mimics the body's own delivery of hormones and decreases the blood-clotting risks that are increased when taking equine estrogens by mouth.

How Much, for How Long?

How long does it take to get some relief from the hot flashes, night sweats, insomnia, and uncomfortable stiff joints? When a woman takes hormones for the first time for menopause symptoms, doctors see several different patterns.

- Moderate doses at 7 weeks—About half of women are completely symptom-free.

- Moderate doses at 14 weeks—More than 9 out of 10 feel fine.

- Highest dose at 2 weeks—Women often get relief from their symptoms. However, the price a woman may have to pay for early relief is some soreness in her breasts that is similar to the soreness she may have had in younger years right before her period.

- Drawbacks to highest dose—Another group of women find that these higher hormone levels make them anxious. So the choice of how quickly to initiate hormone therapy is definitely a personal decision.

My opinion is that hormones are forever. It is the highest standard of care to respond to the needs of women who are symptomatic. When men, for one reason or another, have their testicles removed, they're instantly placed on hormones for the rest of their lives. There is no age at which a doctor would tell a man he no longer needs testosterone. Hormone prescribing for these men is simply the standard of care. Why not the same approach for women?

In the discussion over bioidenticals, no one has mentioned the fact that men have been using bio-identical testosterone for more than 30 years in the patch, without a word of controversy. In contrast, consider the amount of public comment estrogen has engendered.

Using Bioidentical Hormones

Bioidentical estradiol, progesterone, and testos-terone have exceptional track records for safety and are wonderfully effective. You can use them to resolve the symptoms of menopause, support your well-being, and regain your hormone balance.

Estrogen

Estrogen is the gold standard of treatment for hot flashes, insomnia, vaginal dryness, and mood changes associated with the onset of menopause. There is no herbal product or drug formula on the market today that has nearly the broad-spectrum efficacy of estradiol. Neither medications such as antidepressants nor herbal therapies such as St. John's wort or black cohosh have proven to be as effective in double-blind studies. Some herbal therapies also have significant side effects as well as contaminants, and can interfere with normal hor-mone actions.

Problems/Symptoms That Estrogen Fixes:

- Improves sleep disorders, especially awaking in the middle of the night

- Resolves hot flashes
- Often eliminates mood swings and meno-pausal depression
- Reduces the tendency toward weight gain
- Improves dry skin, thin skin, and loss of elasticity
- Restores vaginal tissue strength, elasticity, and resistance to infection
- Cures vaginal atrophy
- Enhances sexual lubrication
- Helps cure low libido and painful inter-course
- Restores strength and elasticity of bladder and urethra
- Reduces risk of urinary tract infections
- May help overcome incontinence
- Decreases joint stiffness and pains
- Prevents osteoporosis
- Reverses bone loss, restores bone strength

Slow-Release Bioidentical Estradiol Products:

- Skin patches applied weekly (Climara) or twice-weekly (Vivelle Dot)
- Vaginal ring, which provides estradiol to the entire body, changed every three months (Femring)
- Vaginal ring, with localized effects that sup-port sexuality and improve bladder function (Estring)

- Vaginal tablet (the size of an aspirin), used twice a week (Vagifem)
- Gel for daily delivery to thigh (Divigel)
- Estradiol spray (Evamist)
- Estradiol in oral tablet form (Estrace)

Creams and Gels:

- Estradiol vaginal cream (Estrace)
- Compounded gel or cream (non-FDA certified) which provides estrogen to the entire body

Plant-Based Conjugated Estrogens

Plant-derived conjugated hormone mixtures, marketed widely with excellent FDA safety data, are sold under many brand names including EstraTab, OrthoEst, and Menest. They come in a variety of dosages and Cenestin and Enjuvia are available in a slow-release form that almost imitates the smooth natural blood levels provided by patches and rings. These are real problem-solver estrogens for women who still don't feel perfectly balanced with bio-identicals alone. Many women have such a positive experience with these conjugated mixtures of estrogens that they don't want to change.

The conjugated estrogens were designed specifically to imitate Premarin because Premarin was so successful in treating menopausal symptoms. The plant-derived conjugated estrogens (see list) are similar to the mix of estrogens in Premarin that relieve symptoms, but do not contain the hundreds of other compounds found in Premarin.

For women who find that bioidenticals are not the ideal match for their body chemistry, the plant-derived mixture of conjugated estrogens seems to provide the missing magical ingredients. It is a bit of a mystery, but we are lucky to have so many options available to us. The major ingredient of the plant-derived conjugated products is Estrone (E1), and the liver converts it as needed to estradiol (E2). Estrone acts as a reservoir for estradiol in the body, helping us keep our hormones on an even keel, even if we forget to take a pill now and then.

Estrogen and Testosterone Combined

There is one product in the United States made from plants that contain both estrogens and testosterone. It is called Estratest and is available in full strength and half strength. It is also available as a generic, which is FDA-approved. The form of testosterone incorporated in this supplement is not strictly bioidentical, but it works very well for many women. It contains methyl-testosterone, a synthetic compound that was made to protect the liver and slow the metabolism of testosterone after it has been absorbed through the GI tract. There are both advantages to this methylated form of testosterone and possible disadvantages, and the response is always unique to each woman's needs.

Progesterone

If you have a uterus, cyclic or continuous progesterone should be taken. Oral forms of progesterone are used by about 90 percent of women taking this hormone. However, those who experience PMS-like symptoms with this oral form usually prefer to take it vaginally. About 10 percent of women use the gel or the time-release tablets (at lower doses) as vaginal suppositories. All three of these options appear to have equal effectiveness.

Because women usually feel great on estrogen alone, it is the progesterone cycle that is most often forgotten. The dose and frequency of progesterone are adjusted using reference data from research on hundreds of thousands of women. Internists and family doctors find that continuous daily use of both estrogen and progesterone is the safest approach because women with these regimens have the least amount of abnormal or unscheduled bleeding.

Problems That Progesterone Prevents:

- Prevents uterine lining overgrowth (hyperplasia), taken in micronized oral tablets, used cyclically or continuously

- To prevent hyperplasia, vaginal progesterone tablets or gel can be used cyclically or continuously, which prevents a PMS-like reaction

Symptoms That Progesterone Fixes:

- Progesterone tablet, gel, or cream can be used for mood support. Progesterone cream, however, is not effective in preventing uterine lining build-up.
- Provides a calming, sleep-enhancing effect for some women, and is used for insomnia.

Product Types:

- Bioidentical progesterone, taken by mouth, used continuously, or taken cyclically 12 to 14 days a month (FDA-approved, slow-release Prometrium and generics)
- Vaginal bioidentical progesterone gel (but not cream), has been proven to reduce uterine lining thickness. It comes in pre-packaged applicators (Crinone).
- Progestin skin patches (non-bioidentical synthetic) combined with bioidentical estradiol (Combipatch and ClimaraPro)
- Oral progestin (non-bioidentical combined with bioidentical estradiol in slow-release tablets (Activella and Angelique))
- Oral progestin (non-bioidentical) combined with bioidentical estradiol in slow-release tablets (Norethindrone)

Side Effects and Cautions:

- In cream form, progesterone is not effective protection against endometrial overgrowth
- Progesterone sublingual tablets are not effective for endometrial protection from overgrowth
- May cause benign breast tenderness similar to menstrual symptoms (lasting 7 to 10 days)
- PMS symptoms may occur when taken by mouth
- Depression is a side effect for some women
- Light bleeding or spotting can occur when taken 14 days a month
- Higher blood triglycerides and inflammatory markers with progestin (MPA) (Provera and PremPro)

Testosterone

Testosterone levels actually begin falling slowly from a woman's mid-30s on, so by the time of menopause they may be 20 to 30ng/ml. Testosterone can be given safely through the skin as a gel or cream. The body's own testosterone production can also be promoted using the precursor DHEA, which the body safely converts to testosterone. The ovary and adrenal glands are both equipped to do this bio-conversion. The testosterone patch for women (Intrinsa) is available in E.U. countries, but not yet FDA-approved in the United States. Benefits of testosterone include improvement of dry skin and the thickening and strengthening of skin and muscle tissue. Night sweats often resolve with the addition of a small dose of testosterone.

Problems/Symptoms That Testosterone Fixes:

- Low libido
- Poor sexual response
- Dry vaginal tissue
- Dry skin anywhere on the body
- Decreased capacity to build and maintain muscle mass
- Need to burn fat stores
- Sleep problems despite adequate estrogen
- Night sweats
- Vulnerable, non-assertive moods

Product Types:

- Transdermal cream or gel, applied to wrists, pubic skin, or vaginal area
- Option to use precursor, bioidentical DHEA rather than compounded testosterone hormone products

Cautions:

- Taken orally, some increased risk of benign liver tumors
- T-patches for men are 10 times too strong for women

- Too much testosterone causes loss of hair from the scalp, the development of unwanted body hair, and acne rash

These lists cover the most widely used products and offer general guidelines you can use to open a discussion with your provider. More exhaustive lists of products are published on the NAMS website.

Charting Your Course

Be sure to set up a follow-up appointment to fine-tune your hormone balance, within one to three months of your initial consultation. At that follow-up visit, plan to review your symptom list and your treatment goals. This is also an opportunity to create an ongoing follow-up plan. You'll want to be sure to mention any new health concerns that may have come to your attention since that initial visit.

Most women find it very satisfying to regain a sense of control and mastery over their own lives. In terms of hormone prescribing, we now have the benefit of 30 years of state-of-the art science and life-changing medical discoveries. These discoveries have been translated into practical tools that we can use to help us enjoy safer, healthier, and fuller lives.

Sleeping Beautifully

In This Chapter

- Avoiding insomnia, low neurotransmitters, and muddled moods
- Pinpointing your sleep issues
- Using practical strategies to get a good night's rest
- Relieving hot flashes with estrogen and lifestyle

As an OB/GYN, the menopausal women I see are often sleeping poorly and racked by hot flashes. At this point in their lives, they worry that they've lost their drive and sparkle. It's reassuring to know that with the development of bioidenticals, there are many safe, effective hormone products that can rebalance a woman's hormones and relieve these miserable symptoms.

Why Sleep Matters

When a woman tells me she's waking up every night at 3 A.M., drenched in sweat from hot flashes, as a physician I consider this situation a four-alarm fire.

Sleep is not a luxury. Restorative sleep re-establishes healthy levels of brain chemicals that are essential to your memory, moods, and focus. On the other hand, chronic insomnia can gradually erode your health.

Without quality sleep, the neurotransmitters can get progressively more depleted, until it becomes difficult to function. Yet some women go without quality sleep week after week, and sometimes year after year. It's not unusual for patients to tell me, "After menopause, my mother never really got another good night's sleep again." Yet it doesn't have to be that way!

Chronic sleep loss has the same negative effects as high alcohol blood levels that exceed legal limits. Your reflexes and your ability to think on your feet in an emergency depend on a good night's sleep. We know that sleep makes a difference, because recent laws addressing sleep deprivation in truck drivers have resulted in fewer traffic accidents.

Insomnia may begin even before menopause, triggered by the initial drop in your hormone levels, often just in the few days before your menstrual period. If you're struggling with insomnia, you may not realize that the underlying cause is the wild ups and downs of your hormones (especially the downs). Yo-yoing hormones can definitely interfere with healthy sleep.

Troubleshooting Sleep

Sleep specialists divide these disorders into several different patterns. Many women experience one of these issues when their hormone levels drop. Your hormones make important contributions to your quality of sleep, how deeply you sleep, and whether or not you dream. We need all the different stages of healthy sleep to be alert and composed.

Can't *Get* to Sleep?

Some women have difficulty getting to sleep in the first place. Anxiety, worry, or financial stresses that they take to bed with them can make it difficult to fall asleep. The causes of this type of insomnia are sometimes complicated, so this pattern is rarely treated successfully with estrogen alone.

Waking Up at 3:00 A.M.?

Most menopausal women can *get* to sleep just fine, but wake up and can't get *back* to sleep. Other women find that they wake up, off and on, through-out the night. They may awaken at 2:30 or 3:00 in the morning and struggle to finally get back to sleep at 5:00 A.M. If you have to get up at 7:00, the result is an absolutely raunchy night of sleep and the recipe for a disastrous day.

Waking up in the middle of the night (nocturnal awakening) is a classic pattern characteristic of hormone imbalance in menopause. This type of insomnia is not usually caused by anxiety or a racing mind. When women wake up with these low-estrogen events, they feel incredibly awake and alert. There is no sense of being sleepy or drowsy, and because it's not easy to fall asleep again, it's a temptation to get up and get something done.

Three nights of this is all you should tolerate before doing something about it. It is among the easiest types of sleep problem to cure, and not dealing with it can quickly compromise your health. The simplest solution is to try a little estrogen support to see if that addresses the underlying cause.

Struggling with Sleep Apnea?

Sleep apnea involves difficulty breathing while one is sleeping. As a result, there's less oxygen in the blood, and quality of sleep definitely suffers. One of the primary causes of apnea in midlife is weight gain that impinges on the airway. This is another issue that ties back to hormones. Women without hormone support tend to gain more weight than those who use hormone replacement. That extra weight is often the cause of apnea, so taking the weight off is the best permanent solution. A good sleep center can diagnose your problem and provide you with additional options, including short-term approaches so you can get a good night's sleep while working on the weight.

Sleep Solutions

The simplest strategy for most women struggling with insomnia is to try a little estrogen support. Some women find that they also need small doses of other hormones to achieve a balance. The goal is to correct the underlying problem and restore the healthy hormone balance that you had before all this chaos began.

This is a better option than masking the problem with sleeping pills that knock you out and deny you the full, deep sleep you need for true restoration. Rebalancing your hormones will also help restore your entire chemistry, and prevent the possibility of sleeping pill side effects, such as impaired memory, nighttime eating, or sleepwalking.

Hormones: Key Players

There are several hormones that can play a role in sleep, including:

- **Estrogen.** In my experience, the best approach is to use a bioidentical estrogen preparation absorbed through the skin. Estrogen can be provided in a patch, cream, gel, vaginal ring, or tiny vaginal tablet. By providing the needed estrogen, other subtle but profound aspects of hormone balance are not disrupted.

- **Testosterone and** *Dehydroepiandrosterone (DHEA).* Testosterone can help balance the availability of your estrogen in the sleep center of your brain. If testosterone levels are low, the addition of its precursor DHEA, or a compounded bioidentical testosterone gel or cream, can help restore good sleep.

- **Progesterone.** For a small number of women, other hormones may be missing that are crucial to the brain. Progesterone is the most common hidden factor in solving the insomnia mystery. Bioidentical progesterone is sometimes taken at bedtime (either orally or vaginally) to help women stay asleep and feel better rested the next day. If this is the missing element for you, it will help restore your body's chemistry. If it's not, you may be one of the women who doesn't really like the way progesterone makes them feel, with symptoms that resemble PMS.

def•i•ni•tion

Dehydroepiandrosterone (DHEA) is a steroid hormone precursor naturally produced by the adrenal glands. It's not a hormone itself, meaning that it doesn't have any biologic activity until it is converted by your built-in hormone transformers (special types of enzymes). DHEA matters because it's a step in the process of making your own hormones, most directly testosterone. Because DHEA is produced in the adrenals, chronic stress can drive down the level of DHEA, affecting other hormones as well.

- **Neurotransmitters.** When hormones drop and you find yourself awakening too easily, this often reflects lower levels of the neurotransmitter adenosine (and possibly others). This magical little chemical is essential to healthy memory and mood. During normal sleep, you replenish the stores of glucose in the brain that are later converted to adenosine. Once your hormones are effectively rebalanced, this should enable you to sleep, which will restore adenosine naturally.

The key to midlife insomnia is to proactively resolve it, rather than accepting it as an inevitable aspect of aging. A good night's sleep is an essential ingredient to good health and optimal quality of life at any age. So if you're sleep-challenged, get professional help, starting with a menopausal hormone evaluation, and sleep tight!

Lifestyle Solutions

There are several lifestyle strategies you can use to improve your slumber, including exercise, good nutrition, and a soothing bedtime routine. You want to intervene before those sleepless nights compromise your health.

- **Walking the talk.** There is a major connection between exercise and sleep. Women who initially push past fatigue to get going will find they're rewarded with better sleep. Walking is a great way to get back in the groove, especially fast walking. Yoga and weight training are also good for starters.

- **Nourishing your sleep.** You want to make sure you get enough protein in the evening so you don't wake up hungry. Include foods that are rich in the amino acid tryptophan to help you fall asleep, such as a mini-turkey sandwich on whole grain crackers. Milk can do the trick if you don't have a problem with lactose (milk sugar) or casein (milk protein). You might also try calcium and/or calcium magnesium supplements. Some women find the herb valerian helpful for insomnia.

- **Tucking yourself in.** If insomnia at bedtime is an issue, you'll want to change your schedule and avoid TV or other distractions at bedtime that stimulate a busy frame of mind. Try a warm shower, a bath, or a soak in Epsom salts or minerals just before bed. You might read something soothing after you go to bed, or use a prayer or meditative phrase that calms you and empties your mind.

Just as we create a mellow, sweet mood to put babies to sleep, we need this for our own tranquil slumber.

Too Hot to Handle

Hot flashes are another symptom that can wreck a good night's sleep. They often occur long before a woman's final menstrual period. As women inch into menopause, many have brief hot flashes right before their period starts. Sometimes this begins several years before the final period.

Drops in estrogen affect the center of the brain that regulates temperature (the hypothalamus). When these drops occur, that means the mechanism for tolerating changes in temperature is no longer working correctly.

The night sweats associated with hot flashes are different than the kind of sweating experienced in hot weather, which helps to cool us down and makes us more comfortable. Hot flashes induced by low estrogen may cause a cycle of hot skin, sweating, evaporation, and then a clammy chill. Some women even describe them as "prickly." If these symptoms are mild, you can almost ignore them. But when hot flashes occur 10 to 15 times in succession, whether they're in the middle of the night or the middle of a sales meeting, it can be extremely distracting.

What specifically causes hot flashes is still a mystery, but we do know that hormonal change is the trigger.

Try a Little Estradiol

The first logical step in resolving these symptoms is to take a trial course of bioidentical estrogen. Research shows that for the majority of women, more than 97 percent of the symptoms of hot flashes are resolved with estrogen therapy. Often addressing hot flashes and night sweats can really improve sleep quality.

For a few women, estrogen isn't the whole story. In that case, the next step is to pay attention to symptoms that suggest low testosterone, such as continued hot flashes despite estradiol at adequate levels. Other signs of woefully inadequate testosterone include dry skin, lack of interest in sex, and lack of progress in weight training. Testosterone helps generate estrogen in the brain where it needs to be to cure hot flashes. Resolving these issues often gains new respect for testosterone. Women are finally able to "get off the dime" with their exercise program and start adding some muscle instead of extra pounds. Remember that testosterone can also help free up estradiol to do its magic. So either hormone could be the key to a good night's sleep.

Upgrade Your Cuisine

There are some simple changes in your diet that can make a big difference in reducing hot flashes and insomnia. The major ones are sugar, alcohol, and protein. Try changing just one factor at a time so you can see what makes the greatest difference.

- **Avoiding sugar.** Cutting out sugar definitely helps reduce hot flashes. You also want to go easy on any kind of simple carb that spikes your blood sugar. The trick is to find other foods that please you and satisfy your hunger. (You can use the Glycemic Index to help you figure out which foods support stable blood sugar. Many women also find the Index useful for weight loss. See www. DrRicki.com.

- **Increasing protein.** You want to get enough protein in your diet to restore your brain chemistry. Protein-rich foods such as turkey actually provide the raw materials that your body converts into neurotransmitters.

- **Minimizing alcohol in the evening.** Alcohol often contributes to hot flashes. Many women find that when they eliminate the glass of wine at night, they also get rid of their hot flashes. One glass of wine gives them a few hot flashes during the evening, and two gives them intrusive night sweats.

- **Cutting down on spicy foods.** Some studies have found that spicy foods can trigger hot flashes. By tracking just one of these factors at a time, you'll be able to see more clearly whether this is an issue for you. No need to avoid spices if they're not a problem.

Take a little extra time to actually look at a few new recipes or check out food magazines to see what appeals to you, and then shop for those new ingredients. Boring is not what makes food fun or interesting. We need variety.

Need Sleep? Work Out, Chill Out

Next to supplementing estrogen, aerobic exercise is the best way to decrease the frequency and severity of hot flashes and improve the quality of your sleep. Aerobics change brain chemistry, so they're useful for supporting good moods, better focus, and more energy. In fact, aerobics are so effective in reducing hot flashes that researchers now have to control for the effects of aerobic exercise when they design research studies. Some women believe that they're just not the kind of person that likes to sweat. But when they finally try it, they are amazed at the difference it makes. It just takes a 20-minute commitment to "feel good, and look good."

The trick is to really get oxygen pumping and work up a healthy sweat. This will increase your levels of neurotransmitters and usually give you the relief you need.

- **Oxygen.** When you exercise, you want your lungs working at maximum capacity, to raise the level of oxygen in your blood.

- **A healthy sweat.** The more you sweat with exercise, the fewer hot flashes you'll have, night and day.

- **Neurotransmitters.** Improving neurotransmitter levels seems to reduce the frequency and severity of hot flashes.

How much exercise and how often? You want that magic minimum 20 minutes a day times 7. That adds up to 140 minutes a week. Work up to the recommended heart rate for your age and weight. It's more important to do a little every day than do an hour twice a week. You want to be free of hot flashes every day, not just the 24 hours after you exercise.

Regaining Your Balance

Your body always seeks a natural balance. You can support this process by restoring your hormones and providing the essential nutrients you need through food and supplements. Other important lifestyle factors include a good night's sleep and daily exercise. Once you have these elements in place, your body will be able to maintain more even levels from day to day. Bioidenticals can be a key factor in restoring this inner balance.

Chapter 7

Taming Rollercoaster Moods

In This Chapter

- The crucial link between low estrogen and low moods
- How less sugar and more protein can improve your mood
- Why exercise provides double the benefits for mood
- When medication becomes important, and when to see your doctor
- How midlife can become an opportunity for growth and true liberation

If you're feeling mood-challenged, what's triggering your moods? Is it your yo-yoing hormones or the unnerving symptoms of menopause? Are you miserable because you haven't had a decent night's sleep or because you're feeling a little dumpy? Or is it the stress of looking in the mirror and seeing your mother's face? It's no wonder that you may be feeling down. Moods are like a puzzle with many pieces—and although some seem to be guided by mysterious forces, others are clearly under our control.

Chasing the Blues

The Problem	The Solution
Up-and-Down Moods	Supplement estrogen (and maybe progesterone)
Blood Sugar Swings	Cut down on carbs and sugar Increase protein Limit alcohol (especially at night)
Lethargy and Fatigue	Increase aerobic exercise Daily strength training
High Stress	Good stress management Mind-body and relaxation techniques Get more sleep (see Chapter 6)
Brain Fog	Stop multi-tasking Get your hormones checked

Tackling Depression with Hormones

There are three key aspects of lifestyle when it comes to mood: hormones, exercise, and nutrition.

1. Of these, hormones are actually the simplest for a physician to figure out, and the rest are up to you. Hormones influence mood for about 70 percent of women. In menopause the vast majority of women find that their moods are improved by taking estrogen.

2. Joyful exercise can also help you recapture a surprising amount of mental and physical energy—whether you're doing Pilates or tai chi, running, or just walking the dog.

3. Another good strategy is to nourish yourself with great food.

Clearly, genetics are an important piece of the puzzle too. Women with a strong family history of depression are more likely to experience blue moods. But we now know that you can influence many aspects of your genetics, through your lifestyle and health behaviors. If you have the genetic risk for a mood disorder, you'll probably find it encouraging to know that hormone supplements can usually restore balance to your hormone levels *and* your moods.

 Hormone Tips

Some women consider themselves to be at the mercy of their hormones. From their first bout of PMS and teen depression to the post-partum blues, they've always been "hormonally challenged." For most of these women, the low estrogen of menopause results in low mood or frank depression. Restoring hormones to pre-menopausal levels at the earliest opportunity can be a lifesaver and can avoid the risk of deeper, more serious depression.

It doesn't seem fair, but women who've had the most intense PMS or PMDD (pre-menstrual dysphoric disorder) when they were younger tend to have a higher incidence of depression in menopause. The good news is that women who struggle with depression are often very responsive to hormone therapy and see improvement with a low dosage of estrogen.

If you're feeling blue and detached from your family or friends, mention this to your care provider. Explore alternatives for treating your mood. Good options include a little estrogen, better nutrition, more exercise, and medications such as antidepressants.

Food and Mood

The relationship between food and mood has been confirmed in scientific terms over the past two decades. We now know that it's important to assess your nutrition and see if that's adding to your stress or helping to relieve it. There have been a great many books on the subject, and the Resources section includes some of the best.

Sack the Sugar

Low blood sugar can have a drastic effect on our moods. Blood sugar often plummets 1) when you've missed a meal or 2) if you've been overdoing sugar or carbs.

Skipping breakfast can be a double whammy. In Margaret's case, she'd down a cup of coffee and a muffin or a sweet roll on her run to the office. This high-carb/low-protein combo often left her depleted, and by late morning she'd crash. High-carb foods can cause blood sugar chaos, bouncing your glucose up and down, and then leaving you running on empty.

Margaret's symptoms were severe—emotional highs and lows, intense hot flashes, and drenching sweats. Periodically, she'd snap at co-workers, which threatened her job. Her history revealed an incredible addiction to sugar.

Warning Label

When it comes to "sugar," we're not just talking about the sugar you dole out by the spoonful. Sugars are hidden in almost all processed and restaurant foods. From sauces to vegetables, almost everything tends to be laced with sucrose, corn sweetener, fructose, maltose, honey, or maple syrup. Same difference. They all add up to disastrous moods, weight gain, and the potential for diabetes. Be sure to check the carb content (and sugars) on the label of the foods you buy. You may be surprised.

Margaret's lab work confirmed that she had severe reactive hypoglycemia. I explained that unless she stabilized her blood sugar, hormone therapy alone would not resolve her symptoms.

When I saw her a month later, she was amazed by how much better she felt. She'd made a real effort to change her diet, and within 10 days her moods had evened out. She had no more hot flashes, and she felt a sense of control she hadn't experienced in two decades. She confided that the last time she'd felt that good, she was expecting her second child and had cut out all the junk food to have a healthy pregnancy. For those of us who've been pregnant and made an extra effort to eat healthy "for the baby," it helps to get back into this mind-set. Remember that you were once a baby too and deserve the same conscientious and loving care.

Protein = Steady State

Erratic behavior, flashes of anger, or extreme mood swings could also be a sign that you're not getting enough protein. This can make you feel desperately hungry and short fused. What's confusing is that these symptoms could either be hormonal or related to blood sugar. To sort out issues of mood and food, get something to eat that includes protein. If the issue is low blood sugar, that will resolve it for the moment.

The next step is to be sure you get enough protein every day at breakfast and lunch (and dinner, if you have trouble sleeping). You may be able to improve your mood simply by increasing the protein in your diet and cutting down on refined carbs, replacing them with satisfying whole grains (such as hearty, sprouted wheat breads or brown rice) and complex carbs (try baked sweet potato fries). Good protein sources include nuts, soy, eggs, dairy products, sea-food, meat, or poultry. At that point, see how you're feeling and functioning.

Often women who are managing their weight don't seem to get enough protein. In an effort to cut down on the amount of fat they eat, they tend to minimize their intake of protein-rich foods. Low-fat/low-protein diets don't provide the nutrients your body needs to create neurotransmitters such as serotonin. And this can make for low moods.

Exercise: The E-Word

Estrogen alone may not do the job. Women who exercise and oxygenate their blood with aerobic activity for at least 20 minutes a day have higher levels of beneficial neurotransmitters. You've heard about "the runner's high." This is real. Exercise is another way to elevate serotonin, the primary neurotransmitter essential for optimal mood chemistry. Women who are depressed usually have low serotonin, so increasing exercise will raise your serotonin and improve your mood.

There is also the magic of oxygen itself. Your cells work best with optimal levels of oxygen. You want to exercise almost every day and get your lungs working at maximum capacity. And yes, you have to sweat to get there. When that happens, you are actually providing extra oxygen to all the tissues and cells in your body, minute to minute. Best of all, you're supporting more cheerful moods, sharper focus, and higher energy.

Meds for Moods

What if you're feeling stuck? If you've tried adding protein (especially in the morning) and getting more exercise, and you're still blue, the next step is to check your hormones again. When you find yourself with a chronic case of the blues, the blahs, or perhaps a deeper *melancholic depression*, you want to take it seriously. At that point, it's important to talk with your doctor. Some women do best on a prescription of antidepressants during the menopause transition to get jumpstarted. After their hormones are stabilized and they've achieved optimal moods, they can wean off the anti-depressants and continue to enjoy life. At that point, they're ready to function "on their own juice" again. Prescription meds aren't necessarily forever. The question of whether you might need medication for your mood calls for a discussion between you and your care provider.

The first step is to become aware of your moods. To download a useful checklist for tracking moods, see www.DrRicki.com. This easy-to-use list will help you see if your mood is low, and whether that's happening very often. It's important to keep track of how you're feeling from day to day, so you can step back and see if there's a pattern related to hormones or life events.

def•i•ni•tion

Melancholic depression is the term used to describe the inability to feel pleasure, accompanied by insomnia, decreased appetite, or physical agitation. Estrogen often relieves this form of depression. Less common is a psychotic depression, a sub-type of major depression, associated with delusional perceptions, and sometimes par-anoid feelings that others are being overly critical. If severe, these emotional distor-tions can become paralyzing and require more than hormone treatment to resolve.

Challenge or Opportunity?

Aging can be a rude awakening, especially when quality of life is severely affected by abrupt hormone changes. It's a big adjustment for those who've lived on cruise control. For the vast majority of women, menopause requires active attention to better self-care or we just don't feel our best.

Menopause can also be stressful for women who were strikingly beautiful in their youth. When they hit midlife, they may feel that they're losing their identity. Women who've focused on outer beauty have to make a conscious shift in their values if they're going to feel fulfilled and happy as they age.

Depression and Dementia

Some women just get the blahs. They don't seem terribly depressed, but aren't excited about anything, either. This can be a mild form of depression, and it's important to recognize it and take steps to resolve it.

In general, women whose depression is not recognized and treated appropriately have higher rates of dementia. Those who drag through the years after menopause feeling less optimistic and less energetic are found to have a higher rate of Alzheimer's. So don't neglect your mood. It may be a message to you from your body that needs attention. The good news is, when depression is treated, the risks are greatly reduced.

Liberation

When you're at this stage, life is more about feeling good and looking your best. You're not going to look 25. But who would want to be 25 again and have to go through the struggles of the 30s and 40s? When we just focus on the outer surface appearance, we tend to forget all we've learned and the wealth of experience we now bring to our lives and those around us.

This can open the door to other opportunities. I call it "soul work." You are liberated from competing on other stages, in other arenas. Now you can do your own soul work. This offers infinite possibilities and new opportunities. Ultimately, there really is no stopping point.

The Skinny on Weight

In This Chapter

- The connection between your hormones and your weight
- The practical steps you can take to avoid diabetes
- The way to lose weight without deprivation
- The big payoff from a little exercise

This chapter gives you the facts on what works, what's hype, and what's not. The keys include support for your hormones, great healthy food, and easy exercise. This is the winning combination. You're going to be surprised at how good you look and how great you feel.

The Hormone-Weight Connection

After menopause, taking the weight off seems harder. Our hormones are at the heart of this dilemma. When estrogen and testosterone drop, we start losing muscle mass. That means fewer calories burned. So every week, month, and year we put on a few more pounds.

As a result many women become mildly prediabetic (insulin-resistant) and the more weight one gains, the worse that gets. Clearly this is a downward spiral, going in the wrong direction. Many women tell me that they still go to the gym, they don't binge or snack, and yet they're gaining 5 pounds a year. Insight on how this happens—and how you can turn this around—are explained in this chapter.

Don't Blame Estrogen

Women tend to blame estrogen for weight gain during menopause. Yet studies show that women who are *not* taking estrogen weigh about 8 pounds more after five years of menopause than those who *took* hormones. We have proof-positive confirmation of this, complete with the telling photographs. MRI images show that when estrogen drops, the volume of muscle still *looks* the same. But close-up shots show that the marbling of fat *within* the muscle increases. So lower estrogen literally means more body fat. You can reverse this trend safely with bioidentical estrogen, paired with progesterone if you have not had a hysterectomy.

The Power of T(estosterone)

Why do lower hormones mean more weight gain? When testosterone drops, it's harder to maintain muscle tone or build new muscle. So if weight gain is your issue, it's important to check your testosterone level, as well as your estrogen. The benefits of good hormone balance include optimal weight, improved physical strength, and less risk of injury. (You also need enough protein so you have the raw materials to build sexy muscles.)

Supporting your hormones improves your mood and motivation by boosting testosterone and balancing one of your primary stress hormones, cortisol. This makes most women feel (1) less stressed and depressed, (2) more like taking care of themselves, and (3) extra motivated to exercise. So if weight is your issue, a little bioidentical testosterone can be a helpful addition to your hormone regimen.

The Other T Word: Thyroid

If you're determined to lose weight, you want to stack the cards in your favor. That means figuring out what's causing your food cravings. There are several health issues that can result in big-time cravings. One of the easiest to check is high or low thyroid levels. It can be helpful to see a doctor and get a thorough physical, including blood tests.

The thyroid really sets the pace of your metabolism. It controls how quickly the body burns energy and makes proteins, and how sensitive you are to other hormones. After age 50 you'll want to have your thyroid blood levels checked each year (it just requires a simple blood test). In addition, you'll want to look through your pantry to be sure there's adequate iodine in your diet. Iodine is essential for making thyroid hormone. Sea salt, kelp, and many types of sushi have naturally high iodine levels to support your thyroid.

The Story of Insulin

Understanding insulin will make it easier to manage your weight. Insulin's job is to get the blood sugar (glucose) out of your blood and into your cells—into muscle cells where it can be burned right away as energy or into fat cells where it is stored for future use.

Insulin to the Rescue

Insulin is mainly called into play whenever we eat foods high in carbohydrates. Carbs are a class of foods that contain either sugars or starches, or both. Here, sweets or highly sweet-and-starchy foods are described simply as high carb foods.

For example, breakfast foods and beverages that are high carb include coffee with sugar, donuts, muffins, sweet rolls, sweetened cereals, pancakes and syrup ... you've already got the picture. But carbs are also hidden in a glass of orange juice, *un*-sweetened cereals such as cornflakes and puffed wheat, and energy bars that contain a high level of "sugars." Here's a look at their effect on our bodies ...

Whenever we eat a high carb food, it quickly spikes blood sugar. The sweeter the food, the higher our blood sugar rises. If it keeps going up, we'd pass out. Eventually we'd go into shock and then into a coma. So the body goes into a little crisis. To avoid passing out, our bodies produce extra insulin. The insulin "grabs" the sugar molecules, pulls the sugar out of our bloodstream, and quickly hides it. Where? Our hiding place is like a money belt, in the tissues right around the waist.

Where Food Cravings Come From

When insulin pulls the blood sugar (glucose) out of the bloodstream, most of that glucose is deposited on our belly, in fat cells. That belly fat (stored under the abdominal wall) takes on a life of its own. As larger and larger amounts of belly fat get deposited, it creates a mass of tissue that functions almost like a separate hormone organ, with its own metabolism. The cells in this fat cause a number of harmful effects. They ...

- Can drive intense food cravings, especially for carbs.
- Drain our energy.
- Interfere with testosterone production.
- Produce "bad" estrogen.

This fat tissue also becomes a major source of estrogen. Only this is sometimes called the bad estrogen, because it causes an imbalance in the different forms of estrogen in the body. It can also compete with the good estrogen (estradiol) in the brain, causing low moods.

In Catherine's case, she originally wanted to try menopause without HRT. But she found that she put on quite a bit of belly fat. She began reconsidering her decision and wanted her baseline hormone levels tested. The result? An estrogen level of 32 *without* HRT (this estrogen was produced solely by her own belly fat). Unfortunately, it (1) raised her level of estrone, causing an imbalance of her natural estrogens, and (2) put her at risk of cancer because she wasn't taking progesterone. (As mentioned earlier, in women with a uterus, estrogen always needs to be opposed with progesterone.) Working together, we developed a hormone and weight-loss plan that included walking and swimming. For Catherine, things are definitely looking up.

Spare the Insulin!

This kind of negative cycle can be reversed by cutting way back on sugar and super-starchy foods, the bad carbs that make you chubby. Those are the foods that spike your blood sugar and require insulin to bring blood sugar back in balance. An amazing number of basic comfort foods are high carb, from graham crackers and peanut butter and jelly sandwiches, to raisins and rice cakes. Oh, and did we mention that all these foods, by definition, make us chubby?

However, there are many *other* foods that require very little insulin—they're lower in sweets and starches, and support more balanced blood sugar. These foods are described as "insulin-sparing" because when you eat them, your blood sugar never spikes. Instead, there's a nice easy rise, and then a gradual decline in blood sugar.

"Dieting" Without Deprivation

The good news is that there are many delicious foods that hardly need any insulin at all. So you can eat them and give your pancreas the afternoon off while you go through the day on cruise control. Great foods that only require minimal insulin (and don't cause weight gain) include:

- Fresh fruits such as strawberries, blueberries, raspberries, cherries, peaches, plums, apples, pears, oranges, grapefruit, and tangerines
- Fresh salad veggies such as lettuces, fresh herbs, tomatoes, sweet red and green peppers, cucumbers, avocadoes, scallions, and celery
- Nonstarchy veggies such as zucchini, green beans, asparagus, broccoli, fresh peas, and onions
- Whole grains such as oatmeal, whole wheat products, brown rice, and wild rice
- Complex carbs such as sweet potatoes and yams, black beans, kidney beans, and split peas
- Proteins such as nuts, seeds, soy, tofu, eggs, yogurt, cheeses, and other dairy products
- Fish, seafood, chicken, turkey, and meats

For a full copy of the Glycemic Index, see www. DrRicki.com.

You can introduce this approach using the South Beach Diet, with a two-week jumpstart by eating salads and low carbs. This can be an excellent way to cut food cravings.

Another approach is to transition to foods that are *moderate* on the Glycemic Index without cutting back on what you eat. This can be useful if you're cooking for a spouse and/or kids. Then you'll want to experiment a little to find their favorite foods on the Index.

Making Good Choices

When you eat whole, fresh foods, by definition they're high in nutrients and fiber. This means far fewer empty calories. It also means fewer food cravings, because you're giving your body what it needs. Using a tool such as the Index, you don't have to cut back on what you eat. You can simply substitute healthy choices in place of the foods that aren't as good for you.

On the other hand, prepackaged foods are a reality in modern life. Just be sure to read labels. Moderate the carbs, minimize the sugars, and get enough fiber and protein. For example, substitute a piece of fresh fruit (that's low on the Index) for that prepackaged orange juice in the morning. The O.J. is virtually pure sugar. Or instead of the juice, have a fresh tangerine, a peach, some strawberries, or a juicy apple.

Motivation and support are other key elements in losing weight. If your goal is good weight management, consider joining a weight-loss program such as Weight Watchers or Jenny Craig, attending a group such as Overeaters Anonymous or Food Addicts, or working with a health coach.

The short list is here:

- Don't forget the hidden calories and carbs
- Increase protein
- Include healthy fats
- Drink eight glasses of water a day
- Burn more calories than you consume

To look good and feel good, start with the right information and make a commitment to loving self-care. Balance your hormones and try to make healthier little choices each day.

Skip That Second Helping

Weight gain creates a wicked domino effect, so you want to find every way that you can to turn this around. Prediabetes (insulin resistance) becomes diabetes if it's not reversed. That paves the way for diseases that you don't want, such as high blood pressure, heart disease, stroke, and cancer. Eating foods that are insulin sparing can reduce or reverse this tendency and avoid the need for oral medications to lower blood sugar. Who wants to use medication for something you can actually prevent?

With balanced bioidentical estrogen and testosterone, it's now possible to move your life in the right direction. But your hormones can't do it alone—you've got to do your part, too.

Hormone Tips

Think in terms of baby steps. If you lower your calorie intake by just 200 calories a day, here's what happens over a year:

200 fewer calories every day × 365 days = 73,000 fewer calories of fat stored in your body

Divide this by 3,600 calories per pound of human fat and you get …

20 pounds lost per year!! That's the math! For example, 200 calories = one grande Starbucks whole milk latte. Skip this and try black coffee with a touch of skim milk if you want the java.

Exercise Every Darned Day

Our bodies are designed for action. For millions of years we hunted and gathered our food, constantly on the move in search of enough calories to survive. The past 50 years have changed all this. Food in the United States is plentiful, and it takes very little energy to get it.

Survival always means adapting. If you live in a modern city, it's not always easy to get enough exercise. That means you need to consciously make exercise part of your routine. Delightfully, when we wrap our minds around these bold truths and commit to regular exercise, we start feeling better almost immediately. Most women notice the benefit their very first day back in the gym, on the bike, in the pool, or on the track. You can road test this information for yourself and see the positive results.

The Plan:

1. First, think about your favorite type of activity. Think joyful! What makes your heart sing *and* pump? At a minimum, you want some form of exercise that you don't hate. The key is to keep doing it.

2. Do the calorie-reality check to see how much you'll burn. Choose your shortlist of activities to meet your requirements for aerobics, weight training, and stretching.

3. Now get out your Blackberry, day planner, or calendar. Make a plan to get active. You want a balanced plan of daily exercise, ideally six or seven days a week. Literally schedule the exercise right into each day.

I was intrigued by this patient's story: when Elana's husband joined a weight-loss team at the Y, she felt a little competitive and that jumpstarted her program. She knew that her steady 4 to 5 pounds of weight gain every year was nudging her toward diabetes. So Elana and Bill went on a low-carb, high-protein diet, complete with ample fresh veggies and low-sugar fruits. She made time for 45 minutes of exercise every day, and walked on days when she couldn't get to the gym. Three times a week, she also did a 30-minute cardio followed by 15 minutes of free weights and stretching. In addition, Elana and Bill walked the family dog for 15 minutes every evening. In four months she had lost 12 pounds! Her blood pressure was the lowest it had been in 15 years. "I feel better than any time I can remember since I started law school over 25 years ago!" All good, and feeling better than ever.

Warning Label

It's interesting that women who sleep more tend to weigh less. The key is energy. Data show that people who get enough sleep exercise more. The reverse is true, too. Sleep less, weigh more. And when we're low on energy, we're also more tempted to turn to carbs for a quick fix. Of course that doesn't fix you. It just makes everything worse.

Burn, Baby, Burn (Calories)

Another great way to get rid of calories is simply to burn them. This is where we can really make some headway. Exercise starts burning off fat stores. It also helps tighten and buff our muscles, burning even more fat. You can see that these are clearly steps in the right direction.

Here's the formula: aerobics + weight training = more muscles and fewer pounds of fat. This is another great reason to work off those calories every day. Muscle mass also increases the *rate* at which you burn fat, by turning up the flame on your metabolism. When you strengthen your thighs and buttocks, that muscle tissue itself becomes similar to an engine that burns calories. (It's just the opposite of belly fat!) As you become more buffed and trim, you'll burn more calories all day long. You'll feel stronger, sexier, and have less risk of sports injuries.

Burning Calories with 30 Minutes of Exercise

Moderate Activities	150–350*
Bicycling (5 mph, flat road)	87
Dancing (ballroom)	105
Swimming (crawl, 20 yards/min)	144
Walking (3 mph)	150
Tennis (doubles)	156
Vigorous Activities	**More Than 350***
Tennis (singles)	225
Aerobic dance	273
Bicycling (13 mph)	306
Jogging (10-minute mile)	327
Circuit weight training	378

*Calories burned per half hour

(Courtesy of www.fitness.gov/exerciseweight.html.)

The Healthy Minimum

Getting started is *the* hardest part of exercise. We all can sit back and say, "I'm just not that kind of person—not a gym rat." But if we're going to survive midlife with grace, we need a new M.O.

Here are some suggestions to kick the sedentary habit:

- **Aerobics.** Just 20 minutes of aerobics every day (you need to sweat and get out of breath). Fast walking or cycling is a great way to get your heart rate up without being hard on your knees. Be sure to drink water to wash the *ketones* (toxins) out of your system.

- **Walking.** Just 30 minutes a day, 7 days a week, to build strength and stability, minimize falls, and reduce stress. You can put 2-pound weights in your vest pockets to strengthen your back, spine, and hips.

- **Weight training.** Only 10 minutes, two times a week, using free weights. You can take the 2-pound weights out of the walking vest pockets for five minutes of your walk and get some exercise for your arms, too.

def•i•ni•tion

> When you're exercising and burning fat, your body produces **ketones**. These byproducts of your body chemistry are a good sign, because they signal that what you're doing is working. But ketones are also a drag, because they make you feel sluggish and tired. Be sure you're getting eight glasses of water a day to remove this "sludge" from your system and improve your energy. (You may worry that your hormones aren't working, but it's probably just the effect of the ketones.)

Lisa exercised in fits and starts—she'd never quite found a regimen she could stick to. She assumed that she'd need at least an hour and a half of gym time to "do *the* ideal routine." My suggestion was that she consider a shorter mini-program that she could do every day. The other strategy was to build in some variation that would allow her to do a range of different exercises during the course of a week. This way she worked different muscle groups and also gave her enough variety to keep her engaged. It wasn't a fancy routine but it turned out to be just enough. "Sometimes perfect is the enemy of good." By doing the bare minimum *and keeping it up*, Lisa was able to slowly and steadily lose weight and arrive pain-free at her goal of a svelte figure.

Ideally you want to see a physical therapist before you start exercising again. I've seen women dive into exercise with a vengeance and get injured. But that just delays the opportunity to feel good again. Remind yourself to ease into exercise, because falling estrogen levels increase the chance of injury. They decrease the thickness of cartilage, and cause a loss of joint fluid. This can all gang up on you and put you at risk when you exercise. The goal is to be able to get out of bed in the morning not with a symphony of aches and pains, but with joy and anticipation.

The Winning Combination

Put the odds in your favor. Give yourself a break. Remind yourself that it took you a long time to become 20 or 30 pounds overweight. And don't go on a punishing diet. The research is unanimous—dieting eventually causes *weight gain*, while a healthy lifestyle change results in fat loss and weight stabilization.

So be sure to treat yourself with the same loving care that you give your children, your family, and your closest friends. Then you'll find the energy and the clarity to do the right thing. The turn-around is this … bioidentical hormones. Better sleep. Lower carbs. More energy. Steady weight loss. A grand slam.

Chapter **9**

Nourishing Your Skin

In This Chapter

- The elegant effects of estrogen
- The dynamics of healthy skin
- The best way to protect your skin from toxins
- The hidden messages in bad hair days

One of the greatest complaints I hear from women in midlife is how concerned they are about their skin. They may no longer have a partner or a love life, their sleep may be lousy, or they may be racked by night sweats, but these issues are nothing compared with their distress over changes in their appearance. Each time they look in the mirror, everything else pales in comparison.

If you share this concern, know that supplementing hormones often restores the skin's appearance and resilience. Ask your doctor about a three-month trial of hormone therapy. Women are often relieved to discover the improvement that a low dosage of estrogen can make. In addition to estrogen, you may need to supplement testosterone to keep your skin plumped and hydrated.

Studies show that for women who begin hormone support early in menopause, the composition of their skin remains fairly stable. Menopausal women who supplement hormones, eat a good diet, exercise, and have a healthy lifestyle usually find that their skin does not change much in terms of luster, firmness, or fullness. In addition, newer skin treatments, including the retinoids, clearly reduce the depth of wrinkle lines for many women, especially if they also supplement estrogen.

The Visible Effects of Estrogen

When estrogen levels plummet, the visible impact on the skin can be striking. In fact, the effects are often so dramatic that doctors can usually tell just by looking whether a woman is taking hormones or not. (This has actually been confirmed in research studies!) There's broad agreement among doctors that hormones support *healthier* skin, as well as cosmetic improvement.

The bad news for women is that unless you actually *use* hormone therapy, most of you will develop wrinkles and sagging skin at an accelerated pace after your 40s.

As men age, they are often able to escape the
wrinkled, sagging skin that plagues women after
menopause. Why is this? Guys continue to produce
estrogen and significant amounts of testosterone
until they're well into their 70s (and sometimes
beyond).

At this point, you already know many of the
resources that will help you make the most of
your health and appearance. There's nothing that
enhances your skin like:

- Supplementing estrogen
- Good nutrition
- Exercise and good circulation
- Drinking enough water
- Not smoking

That's the winning combination.

Up Close and Personal

There's more to your skin than meets the eye.
Composed of two layers, the visible outer surface—
the epidermis—is vulnerable to damage from sunlight, pollution, tobacco smoke, harsh soaps, and
the chemicals in cosmetic products. The inner
dermis supports and nourishes the outer layer.

def•i•ni•tion

> The **dermis,** the underlying tissue of the
> skin, regenerates, repairs, and restores
> the outer, visible layer of skin. This inner
> tissue is rich in collagen, which gives form
> and body to the skin. It's also composed
> of elastin fibers, which provide resilience
> and uplift against gravity's pull. Every cell
> in the dermis contains estrogen receptors,
> which explains why the skin's appearance
> is so exquisitely sensitive to estrogen levels
> in the body.

Estrogen and Exercise

Vulnerability to wrinkles and aging doesn't just
affect the outer, superficial epidermis, but also the
deeper inner dermis. The estrogen receptors in
the dermis are endowed with a rich blood supply
that is highly estrogen-dependent. In fact, estrogen
provides the signals that orchestrate healthy tissue
throughout your body. (This is also true of the skin
of your vagina as well.)

When hormone levels drop, bloodflow to the skin
decreases. As a result, all the processes dependent
on good circulation are slowed, including the supply of nutrients and oxygen to the tissues. This is
why women tend to lose the natural glow of their
complexion after menopause. It's also why injuries
often take longer to heal. Slower circulation affects
every aspect of the skin's health and ultimately its
ability to regenerate.

Aerobic exercise can actually make a visible difference in your skin. When you exercise you supply the
skin with additional bloodflow, which creates that
healthy glow. Exercise and hormone replacement are
a winning combination that provide more benefit to
your skin than any cream or lotion on the market.

Don't Be Thin-Skinned

When estrogen levels start to fall, there is a drop
in the production of collagen and elastin within the
inner layer of the skin. Less collagen and elastin
mean thinner skin that is more easily injured. And
the injuries tend to be more severe and slower to
heal. Think of the aging women you have known
and the incredible cuts and bruises that can develop
as a result of trivial injuries. The skin may also
become so thin that it appears translucent or shiny,
because it's slower to regenerate.

Hormone Tips

If you've decided to go on a diet, these
three tips will help. (1) Good skin elasticity is supported by estrogen. Amazingly,
that elasticity enables your skin to shrink to
fit when you lose weight. (2) Lose weight
slowly. This will allow your body the time
to adjust to the changes naturally. (3) Be
sure to exercise, which will help you keep
the tone of your muscles and skin, avoiding a baggy appearance when you reach
your goal.

Hormones, Vitamins, and Skin

You want to provide all the estrogen and nutrients that your skin needs to thrive. Hormone replacement therapy will help you …

- Have fewer wrinkles.
- Avoid the appearance of dry or lifeless skin.
- Prevent thinning of your skin.
- Become less vulnerable to bruising.
- Heal more quickly from injuries.
- Have less inflammation.
- Develop fewer skin disorders.

Testosterone supports estrogen in enhancing skin moisture production and maintenance, which keeps your skin full and juicy looking. However, easy does it. Too much testosterone—or too much too fast—can cause a bad complexion and pimples that could take a couple months to resolve. So start slow, and increase testosterone levels gradually to give the hormone time to work its regenerative magic.

Nutrients that nourish you and support beautiful skin include ample protein, plenty of fresh fruits and vegetables, leafy greens, essential fatty acids, and water (at least eight glasses a day).

Protecting Your Skin

You want to avoid as many of the toxins in your environment as you can. First think in terms of the exposures that you can control, such as your choice of soaps, cosmetics, and sunscreen. Then consider what else you can do to support healthy skin (the most important is not smoking).

Don't Ravage Your Skin

The Concern	The Solution
Low Hormones	Supplement hormones
Lack of Nutrients	Limit sugar
	Increase protein
	Take a good-quality multivitamin
	Limit alcohol
Not Enough Exercise	Aerobic exercise for good circulation
Exposure to Toxins	Use sunscreen
	Minimize air pollution by filtering the air in your home
	If you smoke, get the support to stop
	Avoid harsh soaps, chemicalized cosmetics, and hair removal creams

If you smoke, it can be quite harmful to your skin. No doubt about it. The chemicals that damage your lungs are also directly harmful to your skin. Smoking causes those little wrinkle lines around the mouth due to exposure to toxins in the smoke. In addition, smoking has a hardening and drying effect on the skin. These effects are so prominent, they can actually be measured and have been studied by dermatologists.

As we age, we become more sensitive to these chemical insults, because there's less of a protective barrier between our skin and our bloodstream. It's a double bind. As women become more and more desperate for solutions to aging skin, their skin becomes more vulnerable.

All the conditions that can be harmful to our skin tend to become worse without estrogen. Skin regeneration slows down as you age, especially in women who aren't on hormone therapy. Any condition involving inflammation is going to be much more difficult to heal without estrogen.

Common inflammatory skin conditions include atopic dermatitis, dandruff, eczema, skin allergies, and connective tissue diseases such as scleroderma. These are typically conditions that result in excessive dryness, itching, and loss of skin elasticity. Many women find these conditions so uncomfortable that they are often motivated to try hormone support.

In addition to increased inflammation as we age, we're all at greater risk of skin cancer. Conclusions from extensive research suggest that estrogen tends to inhibit the growth of skin cancer, which may explain why women develop fewer melanomas than men. Whether you take estrogen or not, it is very important to have a dermatologist or your family doctor periodically look over your entire body, front and back (and even your toes!). You should also look yourself over carefully once a month when you do your breast exam, to note any areas where there are skin changes. Make it a point to report these to your health-care provider. And if you don't like wearing hats, be sure to use sunscreen on your face.

Hair and Nails!

It's getting dry, it's breaking off, it's falling out. The tendency for thinning hair can be genetic, inherited from your mother, father, or grandparents. But you can still have healthier hair by paying attention to your hormone levels, your nutrition, and your lifestyle.

What contributes to those bad hair days when we feel stressed or wired and our hair really shows it? Hair is an amazing barometer that can reflect low estrogen, testosterone, or progesterone, and also high or low thyroid levels. In addition, an imbalance of certain minerals can cause hair loss—too much mercury, too little iron (anemia), or low zinc or magnesium. Hair loss can also be caused by stress or rapid weight loss.

Hair is still a medical mystery. But if you pay attention to how you feel, the messages from your hair can be very empowering. (You can't personally do much about the economy or global warming, but you can take your health into your own hands and optimize it.) Whatever motivates you to take better care of yourself is a gift. Just go with it and don't judge it.

Your nails, like your hair, reflect messages from your body. We now know that weak, peeling nails often indicate imbalances in body chemistry, such as low vitamin D, not enough calcium, lack of protein, or low estrogen. There are a few lab tests that can be helpful in figuring out what's going on. Nail and bone health are both influenced by the same factors. What's good for one improves the other.

- Ask your doctor for a bone density test, as well as a lab test for vitamin D blood levels. Women with weak, peeling nails often have lower bone density than they should. You'll also want to get your thyroid and calcium levels checked, because they're important for strong bones and nails, too.

- To balance out your protein level, just memorize good sources of protein and figure out your favorites. Quality proteins include nuts, seeds, soy, dairy, eggs, fish, seafood, chicken, turkey, and lean meat. For most women, protein is important at breakfast and lunch. If you have insomnia, include ample protein at dinner as well.

You Are the Star of Your Life

If you look at the lifestyle of movie stars with staying power, such as Gwyneth Paltrow and Julia Roberts, by many descriptions they're exceptionally health conscious. They want to optimize the instruments of their employment, which are their bodies and their faces. It's encouraging to know that to varying degrees, optimal health and beauty are available to all of us.

Chapter 10

Sex Life Rx

In This Chapter

- Prescription for a rewarding relationship
- Estrogen *is* the key to good sex and intimacy after 50
- Practical tips and great products
- Help for infections and irritation
- Better solutions for good bladder health

Here's a gripping story that a patient shared with me recently. "Six months ago, when I first saw you, I thought there was nothing right about my marriage or my husband. Yet within a week of starting the estrogen, I couldn't believe what I had overlooked—how attentive my husband has actually been, and how kind and patient he is. Now, when I look back, I just thank God that this little bit of estrogen has restored my perspective and my marriage."

As a gynecologist, I think it's very important that women at midlife get a hormonal assessment before they get a divorce. How much these symptoms contribute to less joy in the bedroom is anyone's guess. But in my observation, it can be a major factor. Surprisingly, a couple's underlying dissatisfaction is often quite physical in nature. Some of the key issues can be improved tremendously if you identify each of the problems, and address them one by one.

Hormone Tips

How is sexual satisfaction defined? And when does sex become an issue? It's a problem when it's a problem for *you*. There is no other universal definition. When a woman feels that having sex is not satisfying—or when the anticipation or the fantasy is better than the real thing—then you know that sex is a problem. Unfortunately, both perimenopause and menopause tend to have a negative impact on sexual satisfaction. Fortunately, these are issues that can often be successfully resolved.

Relationship Rx

Often women have a tendency to put sex on the back burner. During our busy years building a career or growing a family, life gets in the way of good sex. Unfortunately, just when the kids are leaving home and there is more time for the relationship, menopause can deal the final crushing blow to the sexual relationship. If sex wasn't that great *before* menopause, it can become a low priority afterward. On the other hand, sex can be a source of joy and energy, especially now that the fear of pregnancy is gone.

Warning Label

Once menopause is in full swing, the physical logistics of sex can get dicey. But a woman who has enough self-esteem is usually in a relationship that can handle her feedback, and she'll explain what she's going through to her partner long before things are at the breaking point. That same woman doesn't just laugh off these problems with gallows humor or tough it out—she recognizes her symptoms early, and gets them treated and under control.

The woman who does not feel strong enough to speak up, to take care of things before they're really broken, is more likely to have the relationship end. Once she becomes angry and bitter, it's very hard to put things back together because the couple has been growing apart for so long.

Communication with your partner is always a basic essential. True intimacy grows from this healthy foundation. You can build bridges of trust by sharing information honestly and listening actively. For the majority of women, relationship dynamics are a huge part of "getting in the mood" for sex.

Sex: The Physical Game

Even the lucky women who have actually paid attention to their sexuality still notice that, despite their best efforts, sex just isn't what it used to be. Some find that the time to reach orgasm has become unacceptably long. Others notice that the power of desire gradually slips away and pleasure with it. The mechanics of sex also become more challenging due to back pain, stiff joints, or dryness. Ultimately, enjoyment may decrease to a point where women decide that it's just not worth it.

Vaginal dryness often becomes a major inhibition to satisfying sex after the first year of menopause. In our 20s, 30s, and 40s, the tissue lining of the vagina is healthy, elastic, and moist. Estrogen feeds these lining cells and they actively secrete natural lubricant (a form of mucus) and protective lactic acid that keep annoying bacteria from growing and creating unpleasant odors.

When we no longer have adequate amounts of estrogen, those cells stop producing the essential ingredients for healthy tissue. As a result, the vaginal lining loses its inherent lubrication and elasticity. Often it feels as though the entrance is just too tight to allow for comfortable intercourse.

The causes of discomfort are immediately obvious when we look at these tissues through the microscope. First of all, the vaginal lining shrinks and is only about half as thick as it was before menopause. On closer examination, it's clear that the texture of the tissue has changed, too. When we're younger, this tissue has a quality that allows it to stretch like an accordion, with the dynamic demands of intercourse and childbirth. After menopause, vaginal skin loses these essential "comfort fibers" (elastin and collagen) that enable this tissue to be so flexible. It's no wonder that sex becomes uncomfortable, if not outright painful. This is a situation that tends to gradually get worse; for many women, by the time they've gone without estrogen for five years, they are so dry and atrophied that sex has become an impossibility.

Samantha's case was classic. Three years into menopause, Sam sought out a second opinion for painful intercourse which had not been resolved by the topical treatment suggested by her family physician. One look made it clear that she had severe atrophy of the vaginal tissue and a chronic yeast infection that was causing a great deal of inflammation. Her family doc had treated her for yeast repeatedly, but each time the itching had returned in a week or three. Additionally, whenever she had sex it was painful. She had excess thinning of the vaginal lining and some shrinkage due to the lack of estrogen. The solution: to begin nourishing and healing the vaginal tissue, I prescribed four weeks of topical estrogen to be applied twice a day, plus testosterone cream for the entrance tissue to further support healing. We also decided on a Femring .05 (a vaginal ring with time-released estradiol) to provide estrogen to her entire body. Sam returned with a glowing report. "I can't believe how normal I feel already! Our twenty-fifth wedding anniversary was last weekend and we had a glorious second honeymoon, pain-free!"

Simple Solutions

Glancing at the magazine rack while grocery shopping, we're hit with titles such as "Secrets of Keeping Sex Hot" or "Recipes for Simmering Summer Sex" and even "Hot Bedroom Tips for Today's Woman."

We have the real secrets, because when you get to midlife and beyond, hormones have a lot more to do with sexuality than anything you can buy in the grocery store. Although this isn't about "scintillating secrets," we do have suggestions for a number of great products that are going to give you better sex and intimacy.

Sexual lubricants can be helpful, especially water-based products such as Astroglide or KY-Silk-E, which tend to be moister, stay wet longer, and serve as a better form of lubrication for women. (Do not use Vaseline or KY-Jelly—they are too thick and can lead to irritation.)

Menopausal women who have never had a vaginal birth may experience greater discomfort during sex. When estrogen levels fall, the vagina can become so tight that it is difficult to have intercourse without painful tearing of the vaginal tissue. Sustained estrogen treatment, locally or systemically, is usually very successful, but needs to be used as long as women want to continue having sex.

Simple vaginal dryness is easy to treat. Even women who do not want systemic estrogen replacement can use one of the excellent estrogen products that are now available to address vaginal dryness. Most contain bioidentical hormones and are remarkably effective. Bioidentical estradiol cream is widely available in pharmacies under the brand name Estrace. Additional choices include Premarin Vaginal Cream and Bithena (a plant-based, conjugated estrogen). Regular use of estrogen for localized effects, via a cream, ring, or vaginal suppository, often returns vaginal elasticity to normal pre-menopausal levels within a month or two. Topical use of an estrogen cream also prevents tearing and can make sex comfortable and enjoyable again.

Infections, Irritations, and Annoyances

Women often want to understand the how and why of these annoying vaginal infections that seem to gang up on them after menopause. There are basic biologic reasons for these frustrating little problems. First is the change in the chemistry of the vagina and bladder, due to a drop in the naturally produced vaginal acidity. We're used to thinking of acidity as harmful, but the acidity of the vagina is actually protective. The acid has a health-promoting effect by creating an environment where bacteria cannot thrive. It is this behind-the-scenes acid production by the cells of the vagina that is our first defense against the overgrowth of bacteria. The vagina is really a small ecosystem unto itself.

This delicate balance is very dependent on a healthy minimum of estrogen in the bloodstream. Fortunately, before menopause, most women have a good balance of vaginal flora (beneficial bacteria like acidophilus). The good bacteria actually keep out invading troublemakers such as foul bacteria and yeast. The beauty of hormone support is that when you provide the vagina with sufficient estrogen, you prevent all kinds of vaginal problems, including vaginosis and irritation caused by a harmful bacterial imbalance or yeast. You also reduce the risk of bladder infections at the same time.

Estrogen supplementation also reverses thinning of the vaginal lining by thickening and rebuilding both the inner and outer layers of the tissue. Estrogen therapy promotes a more pleasurable sex life, but also better physical health.

Hormone Tips

Some compounding pharmacies offer estriol cream for women who seem to be unusually sensitive to estradiol products. These appear to be safe but there is no reliable research to define how much estrogen is contained in these products and therefore how long they can be safely used. In contrast, FDA-approved products contain a consistent, predictable amount of estrogen. *There are no herbal products available over the counter that have proven to be as effective as estrogen.*

Inner Health: Urinary Issues

Another benefit of improved vaginal health is better function of the urinary tract. For most women the bladder and the urethra (the tube leading out of the bladder) are noticeably estrogen-dependent. Fortunately, many women do not experience urinary frequency or irritation as they urinate. However, many nagging health problems seem to get worse at menopause and that can interfere with the ability to relax into a fulfilling sexuality.

Infection Mimics

Many women have recurrent or ongoing symptoms of frequent or painful urination, even though they don't have a bladder infection. This is referred to as interstitial cystitis, or IC, which can have a hormonal basis in many women.

The best way to find out if this condition has a hormonal basis is to try estrogen replacement for at least three months to see if bladder symptoms improve. Many women find that the symptoms completely disappear with estrogen's many restorative effects.

Deeper Understanding

A tight, narrowed urethra often leads to more bladder infections. Some women choose estrogen support for this reason alone. Undiagnosed urinary infections can actually become life-threatening in older women, especially in women who do not drink ample amounts of water. Those who have more discomfort with urination avoid drinking to decrease painful trips to the bathroom, and it can pave a path in an unhealthy direction. If you have urinary symptoms, please see a care provider and mention them as a concern.

After estrogen levels are increased with hormone therapy, the urethra and bladder function better. A well-estrogenized urethra is a healthier channel for emptying urine from the bladder, and more resistant to infection. The same is true of bladder health and resistance to disease. Small changes can have a big impact when it comes to these areas of our anatomy.

Regaining Control

Another concern is the sense of not being in control of one's urine. Some women experience this when they cough or sneeze, leaking a little urine. Others find that when they get up from a chair, go up stairs, or laugh heartily, it is difficult to hold their urine. The problem is a loss of strength in the support muscles of the urethra (the tube through which the urine passes) because these muscles are also estrogen-dependent. (Being very overweight usually makes these problems worse.)

Supplementing estrogen can strengthen the pelvic muscles when sufficient systemic estrogen is provided to the entire pelvic floor, including the vagina, bladder, and urethra. Although the research on incontinence and estrogen shows conflicting results, in clinical experience with patients, we find that these treatments make a big difference.

Women who get regular exercise usually have less of a tendency to develop these issues. Yoga and Pilates are excellent exercise practices that add strength to the pelvic floor. In addition, these practices are relaxing, improve posture, enhance orgasms, and are fun to learn and do. Taking a yoga or Pilates class twice a week can make a positive difference.

In terms of exercise, there also is an entire specialty within physical therapy with practices devoted to strengthening the pelvic floor. The first Kegel exercises are now just one small part of this approach, which is known to be of great benefit (for several useful books and websites on strengthening the pelvic floor, see Appendix B). If you are grappling with these issues, you deserve a trial of estrogen and also physical therapy to strengthen the pelvic floor to see if that resolves the problem. Women for whom systemic estrogen is not advised can still use one of the excellent topical treatments that usually take care of this problem without controversy. Only after these approaches have been tried do most gynecologists recommend a surgical approach for repairing urinary incontinence.

You at Your Best

Women are often very self-conscious when talking about these delicate issues. Despite all our years of experience and wisdom, we are not necessarily at ease with our sexuality or areas of our bodies that are intimately associated with sex. Some women seem to feel that urinary dysfunction is a personal failing. Yet often these problems actually have a genetic basis. The strength or weakness of the pelvic floor is actually inherited by virtue of the tensile strength of your connective tissue (which is determined by your genes). The rest relates to lifestyle, obstetric history, and sexual energy and inclination. We need to free ourselves of any blame for these problems. They come with the territory of living longer and being mostly sedentary.

I'll never forget the 84-year-old woman I cared for in my first year of gynecology practice, from whom I learned so much. On her two-week, post-op hysterectomy visit—after a full exam and reassurance that everything was healing beautifully—I asked if she had any more questions. She answered, "When may I *resume* intercourse?" As I was only 30 years old myself I sat up and took a lesson! It had not occurred to me that she was still sexually active in the first place. But to have this burning question on her post-op exam, so soon after surgery, told me that women have quite a lot to look forward to.

May you find your own voice and your own comfort level in terms of sexuality and intimacy. It is a unique human gift to have these spectacular intimate opportunities if we seek them and honor the time and effort to get them right.

Heart and Mind

In This Chapter

- Heart disease or breast cancer—what's your worry?
- Heart-healthy hormones
- Estrogen's exceptional protection against the risk of Alzheimer's
- Surprising safeguards from Parkinson's
- Preventive strategies for depression and dementia

In midlife, many of us find ourselves caring for aging parents who are struggling with heart failure or dementia. This kind of challenge has earned us the label "the sandwich generation." We're pressed between the demands of kids, parents, home, career, self-care, and marriage, if we still have one.

"Aging isn't for sissies." It's frightening for most of us to imagine ourselves in our parents' shoes. Almost every middle-aged woman I see wonders what she can possibly do to avoid her mother's problems. And it's true. There's no denying that aging is a daunting challenge. But at this point in medicine, we now know enough about the prevention of disease to change the course of aging.

Heart disease is the number-one silent killer of women. Survey after survey confirms that women are terrified of breast cancer, but the data show that heart disease is really the greatest threat. The numbers speak for themselves. The yearly deaths for women in 2005 include:

- All forms of heart disease—900,000
- All cancers—about 270,000
- Breast cancer—41,000

def•i•ni•tion

Heart disease describes several conditions in which the heart and blood vessels are clogged with plaque, and can no longer support good circulation. Over time this contributes to high blood pressure and an irregular heartbeat, as well as an increased risk of clotting, stroke, and heart attack. Exercise and even ordinary activities may become severely limited. By the age of 54, one in three American women have some type of problem with their heart. By 75, eight of every ten women have a heart condition.

The Heart of the Matter

Midlife is the ideal time to begin a program to prevent heart disease. We now know how to reverse these trends. So it's a matter of applying what we know. For women, estrogen is often an important piece of the solution, because it helps our blood vessels stay relaxed. In menopause, as estrogen levels fall, there is a tendency to higher blood pressure. Restoring estrogen reverses this trend, lowering blood pressure, improving healthy cholesterol levels, and reducing inflammation throughout the body.

Tammy had a classic family history of heart disease, so she came to see me with questions about hormone therapy when she learned that estrogen could significantly reduce her risk of heart disease.

Both her folks were former smokers, and her dad needed triple bypass surgery after his first heart attack. Her mother had been on meds for years to treat an irregular heartbeat and high blood pressure. Now that Tammy had turned 50, even though she was trim and fit, she worried about the health of her heart. Given her family history, she felt the odds were not in her favor.

If you're fortunate and you've inherited good genes, that's all well and good. But if you're like so many women that have parents such as Tammy's, the genetic risks for heart disease are often carried to the next generation. Research shows that it is possible to "de-program" these genetic tendencies by addressing each of the major risk factors.

How do you prevent heart disease?

- Lower cholesterol
- Maintain normal blood pressure
- Prevent diabetes
- Daily aerobic exercise
- Don't smoke or stop if you do
- Support estrogen levels

Tammy was highly motivated by the problems of her parents, who had been through a series of health crises. In Tammy's case, she'd maintained normal blood pressure and cholesterol throughout her pre-menopause years. Her Mediterranean diet and daily exercise added up to excellent health. After her periods stopped she wanted to add hormone supplements to her program, to help her deal with insomnia (which is often hormone related) *and* also to support her health.

We reviewed the positive effects of estrogen on the heart, blood vessels, and cholesterol. We also looked at the data which showed the importance of starting early for the greatest success in reducing heart disease risk. (Use of estrogen typically lowers these risks by at least one third.) We also discussed the benefits of transdermal bioidenticals in eliminating the risk of blood clots associated with the use of other types of hormones that are taken by mouth.

Tammy's transition to menopause went very smoothly. She tried the support of a tiny low-dose

estradiol patch from her earliest hot flashes until
her menstrual periods started skipping around.
We paired that with bioidentical progesterone, 12
days a month. Given her genetic risks, we periodically check her progress with lab tests, which have
confirmed her good health. Confident that she has
made the right choice, her lab results give her the
reassurance that things are as good as they seem.
On her most recent visit, she said in amazement,
"Menopause has turned out to be easier than I ever
dreamed possible."

Absent-Minded or Alzheimer's?

Emily carried a great deal of anxiety about dementia. A patient in early menopause, her mother had
just been diagnosed with full-blown Alzheimer's.
For Emily, her own brain fog, caused by falling
estrogen levels, was terrifying. "I worry that I'm
becoming like my mother. She's reached a point
where she can't remember anything and seems
spaced out a lot of the time. Now I wonder if my
own mind is slipping away."

When we developed a plan for Emily's care, I
shared the finding that estrogen is highly protective against Alzheimer's, reducing the incidence
by at least 50 percent. We talked about addressing
her sleep first to sustain her focus and her ability
to cope. Then we discussed the details of the long-
term plan to support her in menopause and minimize her risks for dementia.

Curing her sleep disorder was easy. With a daily dose of hormones she began sleeping well again within a matter of weeks. The brain fog was gone by the three-month follow-up visit. Emily chose the combination of estradiol plus progesterone daily because of her history of fibroids and heavy, painful periods, and she said "it worked like a charm." Now that she had confidence her brain was fine, we took a closer look at the important details about hormones, and the long-term health of her mind and memory. There are so many studies that speak to this critical point. In essence, the earlier we start hormones, and the longer we stay on them, the less likely we are to develop Alzheimer's disease.

Research consistently shows that men have lower rates of dementia than women, because men never have the drop in hormone levels that women experience. The women who do as well as men are those who have taken hormones from the first years of menopause and stayed on them longest. The studies indicate that sustained estrogen use is the key. In the research studies, even women who did not exercise but took estrogen from menopause on had a 46 percent reduced risk for Alzheimer's. As menopausal women we have the opportunity to protect ourselves against Alzheimer's with estrogen. This protective effect was first recognized in the research about 10 years ago.

How much of a difference hormones can make depends on other factors in our lifestyle that are totally up to us. There is no pill, patch, lotion, or ring that undoes the harmful effects of an unhealthy lifestyle. The more we commit ourselves to healthy life choices, the better we can expect to do. Our good intentions, put into practice, improve our health and enjoyment of life. Lifestyle really is the key to better health.

Hormone Tips

Estrogen may be the missing piece to the puzzle of memory loss in menopause. Of hundreds of women tested in menopause, not one performed better without estrogen. The majority of women in the studies did better by at least 30 percent in all areas of mental activity when they were using estrogen supplements. It's comforting to know that what relieves our hot flashes and sleepless nights is also good for the mind.

More on the Mind

In Adele's case, her anxiety was driven by her mother's recent diagnosis of early Parkinson's. (I found myself wishing that I could turn back the clock—that we'd had access to the new, safer hormone products 30 years ago, when it might have made a difference for Adele's mother.)

But Adele has her own set of challenges. At 40, she's a busy professional who has also managed to be happily married, give birth to two great kids and launch them off to college, while also being supportive to her mother. As if that weren't enough to deal with, she'd developed fibroids that had grown so large, the best treatment really was a hysterectomy. Because of her fairly severe endometriosis and ovarian pain, she elected to have her ovaries removed at the same time.

Research has found that women who lost their ovaries early and did *not* take estrogen tended to have more Parkinson's disease and other forms of dementia. Fortunately, we know a great deal about the protective effects of estrogen therapy against dementia and Parkinson's.

Recently published studies compared the health of two groups of women: those who had their ovaries removed and those who had not. The women in both groups that did not take estrogen had more Parkinson's and more heart disease. The data show that they also tended to develop these conditions at a younger age.

These studies parallel other data on the protective effects of estrogen for both the brain and heart. For example, images of brain tissue look healthier in the women who took estrogen after menopause, compared with the images of those who did not. Similarly, the blood vessels of the heart itself looked significantly healthier in women who took estrogen compared with those who took no estrogen. This was a finding of the largest study on estrogen to date, the seven-year estrogen-only group in the Women's Health Initiative. The fact that all the women in this study had previously had hysterectomies enabled researchers to see the pure effects of estrogen.

In Adele's case, we discussed the pros and cons of removing the ovaries before natural menopause. To make the right choice, it was important for Adele to know that there is strong evidence on the protective effects of estrogen and testosterone against Parkinson's. So if Adele were to consent to the removal of her ovaries, I wanted to be clear that it was essential she be dedicated to ongoing estrogen and testosterone support. It is of little use to take hormones briefly if your goal is lower risks for long-term health. Adele was motivated and decided to start early and stay on hormones.

Warning Label

Toxic exposure from pesticides can have harmful effects on the brain. Studies have found that Alzheimer's and Parkinson's patients have much higher levels of pesticides in their brain tissue. This is a compelling reason to eat organic foods whenever possible and to use organic products in your home and garden. Many pesticide chemicals are employed for their paralyzing effects on the nervous system of insects and unfortunately these toxins seem to also affect the human nervous system. Pesticide toxins also disrupt human hormone balance by mimicking estrogen.

Dementia and Depression

Many women are surprised to learn that there is a link between dementia and depression. The good news here is that this risk factor is one we can almost always treat.

When Alice was immobilized by depression, everyone was surprised, because she had been highly active in the community. She was a member of the hospital board of trustees and founded a preschool for her grandchildren. But after her husband of 40 years died suddenly of a heart attack, Alice sank into a deep depression. When this condition went untreated, Alice just seemed to disappear into a depressive dementia.

Her daughter Susan (my patient) was entering perimenopause and wanted to do all she could to reduce her own chances of depression and dementia. Of all the frightening considerations women face, dementia and strokes are perhaps their greatest concerns. Dementia is much more likely to develop in women with depression, an increased risk of 30 to 40 percent by best estimates from researchers. The good news is that research also shows a reduction in risk if the depression is recognized and successfully treated.

For Susan, knowing the signs of depression and seeking out professional help early will decrease her own individual risk, so she won't have to suffer her mother's fate. Women who find themselves a little blue or even frankly depressed will feel better in the short-term by addressing and resolving the depression. That also lowers their long-term risk of cognitive loss and dementia.

So don't just put up with the blues. Pick up the phone, call your doctor, and get started on a path toward resolution and treatment if you need it. It's important to look at the risk factors we can modify to lower our risk of disease and do something about those that we can. (Also, see Chapter 7 for more information on managing moods.)

Mental Gymnastics

Estrogen alone can't do the job of protecting us. But lifestyle factors appear to decrease risk for stroke and dementia by about half. Top on the shortlist are daily aerobic exercise, cholesterol levels in a healthy range, and meaningful social connections. Other factors include:

- Supplementing estrogen after menopause
- Staying hydrated
- Good nutrition
- Addressing depression
- Minimizing medication side effects

The aerobic exercise piece is especially important because clearly those who achieve 20 minutes a day of vigorous aerobic exercise have less dementia. They also have less heart disease and cardiovascular risk in general. Eating a low-fat diet appears to significantly reduce the risk of vascular dementia. In addition, a low-calorie diet can be significant in preventing brain atrophy.

Another aspect of reducing your risk for dementia is of course reducing your general cardiovascular disease risk, because at least half the dementias that we see today in older people are the results of a series of small strokes. Be sure to get the support you need to quit smoking if you are a smoker—studies estimate a 75 percent lower risk for heart disease and stroke in nonsmokers.

From Confusion to Clarity

You've had a look at the lives of real women with significant health risks. The scientific evidence makes it clear that many of the diseases of aging can be prevented. At this point, the opportunity for prevention is not just an idea, it is a reality.

12

Changing Bodies, Changing Needs

In This Chapter

- Sustaining your gains
- Meeting your changing needs
- Finding the right balance
- Fine-tuning your program and keeping it going

Our bodies are dynamic and change continually throughout our lives. In this chapter we take a look at how we can keep pace with those changing needs.

The story of bone health serves as a case in point. The best way to achieve optimal health is to look at what we know about the long-term effects of aging on health, *and apply that in the present*. So the ideal personal plan must meet your needs at this moment in time, and also address future risks. Because bone loss affects 80 percent of women by age 75, this is an important feature of every woman's long-term plan and we need to keep an eye on it even when we're young.

More than 85 percent of *osteoporosis* can be prevented by taking hormone supplements. This is the finding from studies involving more than one million women in all major countries of the world. Yet in the United States, due to the breast cancer scares, women still are not using hormone support—even though safer hormone products are now available. As a result, unless we change our approach, one of every two women older than 50 will experience a fracture due to osteoporosis during her lifetime.

Every year, more than two million American women fracture a bone due to osteoporosis, including:

- 300,000 hip fractures
- 550,000 fractured vertebrae
- 1,200,000 other types of fractures

And if these numbers are not frightening enough, 25 percent of the women with hip fractures (one in four) will die within the year following her fracture, due to complications. Women need to listen up, change these horrible statistics, and not become one of them.

When you think about a health issue, it's helpful to understand the human side of an issue by looking at the impact on individual women. Because stories are one of the ways we've always shared ideas, this chapter offers the stories of three different women and the health issues they faced. The stories weave together real concerns and reveal the solutions each one chose. Although the details were specific to these women, the challenges they faced apply to us all.

def•i•ni•tion

> **Osteoporosis** is a bone disease that can be prevented and treated. It involves weak or porous bone tissue, with a breakdown in the structure and content of the bone. This leads to fragile bones, and an increased risk of fractures of the hip, spine, and wrist. Osteopenia is defined as milder bone loss, with bone density that is lower than that found in normal 30-year-old women, but not as perilously low as osteoporosis.

Keeping Your Balance

Whenever we're making health-care decisions that will affect our future, it provides an opportunity for prevention. Today we actually have the data and the understanding to predict the outcome of our choices in advance.

In terms of osteoporosis, if we just "go with the flow" we may wind up in a place we'd prefer not to be, with crumbling bones and frail health. We can counter loss of bone if we are aware of the few crucial actions we must take to rebuild and maintain healthy bones.

I met Ingrid when she was 46, early in her peri-menopause. With a strong family history of breast cancer, she had tested positive for the breast cancer gene. She shared the trait with one of her sisters, her mother, and an aunt. She came to me with issues related to her menopause—she wanted to be able to sleep through the night without intrusive night sweats. Recently remarried, she also wanted to remain sexually active. Her periods had stopped over a year ago, and already she was feeling dry and unenthusiastic about sex.

In addition, she was dealing with asthma, which had gotten worse as she progressed into menopause. She'd been prescribed steroids off and on since childhood to help her breathing. The medication had already resulted in some major bone loss. Steroids clearly increase the rate of bone loss and the risk of a broken bone. The longer the steroid use, the lower the bone density. As a result, Ingrid's bones were 50 percent lighter than those of her sisters. Our goal was to treat her menopause symptoms, start rebuilding her bones, and lower her risk for fractures. Fortunately, estrogen is the ideal choice for all three of these tasks.

To address her breast cancer concerns, Ingrid and I worked with a genetic specialist whose area of expertise was cancer risk genetics. The geneticist shared the data showing that estrogen *lowers* the risk for breast cancer in women in general, including those carrying the breast cancer gene. That was a huge relief.

Ingrid decided on a hormone program that included the bioidentical estrogen ring (Femring) and cyclic bioidentical progesterone (Prometrium). To help her rebuild bone, I recommended ample calcium, vitamin D, and weight-bearing exercise such as weight training. This program supports the health and lifestyle she desires without the symptoms of menopause.

Since then, her follow-up tests for bone density studies show that her bones are getting stronger rather than weaker. Her annual mammograms continue to all be normal and she's thrilled to be symptom-free. As an added bonus, stabilizing her estrogen levels has decreased her frequency of asthma.

Hormone Tips

For optimal bone health, add weight training. Research shows that a year-long strength training program for women after menopause *increased* their spinal bone mass by 9 percent. Women who do not use estrogen or participate in strength training actually experience a *decrease* in bone density from 1 to 5 percent a year. Interestingly, research has shown these same positive results with strength training even in older women (and men) who are 85 to 95 years old, giving us younger women encouragement to get going with the weights!

Fine-Tuning Your Program

Doctors measure patients' successes by good results on their lab tests, yet the right solution is always a balance that includes relief from symptoms, satisfaction with personal issues, and improvement of long-term health. Keep a healthy focus on your goals and readjust your program as your needs change. The other important piece in this balance is active participation in your own self-care.

When Deanne first came to me, she was only 52, but exhausted by a menopause chock-full of hot flashes and migraine headaches. She decided to try estrogen after she learned that for more than half of women, low-dose estrogen in menopause improves migraines. This improvement occurs most often in cases in which the headaches have always been hormonally related.

She also wanted some form of hormone support for her low bone density. Deanna had been a top gymnast throughout high school and college. The most successful athletes, gymnasts, dancers, and supermodels maintain an exceptionally lean body mass to perform with maximum grace and ease. This minimal body fat makes them more agile and lighter on their feet. But women who stay very thin have hormone changes that may stop their menstrual cycles. And these same women often have very low estrogen levels. (In that lean state, the body perceives starvation, so it shuts down fertility, to protect the woman from the stress of pregnancy and another mouth to feed when food supplies are scarce.)

When estrogen levels drop, even at such a young age, it duplicates some of the patterns of menopause. Many young women experience the same bone loss that is caused by low estrogen after 50. Unfortunately, in a young gymnast or dancer, this bone loss may occur at the age of 15 or 16, before her bones have even developed maximum strength.

In Deanna's case, she'd had headaches since college. Although they'd gotten better over the years, with the wild storms of early menopause, she was having a migraine every week. The best way to explore the possibility of improvement would be to try it and find out. Given her low bone density and the impact of menopause on her headaches (and her love life), Deanne was clear that estrogen deserved at least a three-month trial.

The majority of her lab results looked good, so she started on the lowest dose estradiol patch, religiously changing it twice a week to keep her hormone level steady. We chose a low dosage because then she would have the least need for progesterone, which can be associated with headaches in some women. If she needed more estrogen for comfort in making love, we could always increase the systemic estrogen or prescribe a local estrogen cream.

The beauty of Deanne's story also includes our success with her nutrition. Rebuilding her bones meant supporting her calcium supply, so we added calcium citrate, vitamin D, and omega 3 fatty acids (either fish oil or flaxseed oil). I prescribed weight training and of course good hydration along with her exercise.

Five years later, Deanne's bone density is actually better than it was when she was 52. Oh yes, and her migraine headaches are down to fewer than one per year. Fortunately, Deanne began estrogen early enough in the course of her menopause that her skin, bones, and muscle mass have been beautifully supported.

"Self-Care" Is "Primary Care"

Women tend to be natural-born problem solvers. But too often we turn our attention to the needs of others. Menopause serves as a benchmark in time that is undeniable. It makes us sit up and take notice of our own issues. This is a good time to break habits like grab-and-go nutrition, erratic exercise, or doing without sleep.

Warning Label

Don't forget the vitamin D! Vitamin D is a collection of fat-soluble hormone-like molecules produced by our skin when it's exposed to sunlight (without sunblock). Vitamin D_3 (cholecalciferol is the active form) promotes absorption of calcium from food and supplements in the digestive track, and promotes the beneficial re-absorption of calcium into bone tissue. Calcium is the essential raw material we need to maintain our bones and keep them strong. Vitamin D also supports the immune system by promoting anti-tumor activity and other important immune functions.

We need to make a commitment to better self-care. We've done it for our family and friends. Now it's high time we construct a plan to do it for ourselves. The recipe for improvement is simple and it starts with you.

Every Day Is a New Day

You have to sustain a healthy lifestyle. It can't be like a fad diet. It has to be a mature commitment, every delightful day. The most successful women are constantly remodeling, refashioning, and rebuilding their lives as they age. It is inspiring to see these accomplished older women. They provide a vision of what is possible.

We can grow into a healthier future if we keep a "can-do, problem-solving, will-do" attitude. It works best to be optimistic—that's the can-do. The problem-solving means getting good information to support the best solution. And the will-do piece is the commitment to do whatever it takes, to act on what we know. It is in that consistent commitment that we build a foundation for our health, so we can be healthy enough to enjoy life, day to day.

Women have never lived this long before in any numbers, so in a sense we are pioneers, evolving on a learning journey. To experience a long life *with quality of life*, it is essential that we give wise, careful attention to ourselves. As a species we've been here for millions of years, yet few of us have ever experienced growing older before. So we need to bring all our creativity to this new experience, by practicing loving self-care every day.

The most important factor in this success is finding what is sustainable for *you*. There is a solution to meet every woman's needs, to address and master the challenges of healthy aging.

In my practice each day I see women of every age from midlife on, who are aging with grace and vigor. Many have busy successful lives, full-on careers—women from all walks of life, including professionals, educators, and entrepreneurs. I see that we can age differently than our mothers.

I've also had the opportunity of a new perspective, diligently gleaned from the massive scientific research that emerges every month on this topic. I've also witnessed the benefits of this new, safer approach to hormone therapy in thousands of women. They are able to lead fuller, healthier lives than our mother's generation. The majority of these women are also more active and more vigorous than other women their age in the current generation. The fact that I've seen what is possible, not just in a few women but in thousands of women, has been one of my motivations for writing this book.

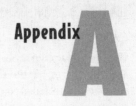

Glossary

androgen Any natural or synthetic hormone with effects similar to those of testosterone.

atrophy Wasting or decreasing in size or thickness of an organ or tissue; a wasting away, deterioration, or diminution. During menopause, these effects are due to decreases in hormone levels.

conjugated estrogen A form of estrogen chemically linked to another molecule that slows activity and metabolism. Conjugated estrogens come in forms extracted from animals, as well as bio-similar estrogens from plants.

continuous combined hormone replacement therapy The daily use of estrogen paired with progesterone or progestin.

cyclical progesterone Giving progesterone on a cycle that replicates a woman's own cycle during her fertile years: 12 to 14 days of progesterone per month.

dysfunctional uterine bleeding Any bleeding that is from the uterus, but not expected.

endometrial hyperplasia Excessive thickening or overgrowth of the uterine lining. Most often the result of an imbalance of the stimulatory effects of estrogen not adequately opposed by progesterone or synthetic progestin. This hyperplasia is a known precursor to uterine cancer, which may be diagnosed by sonogram imaging or tissue biopsy.

endometriosis A common medical condition characterized by growth of the tissue that lines the uterus (the endometrium) beyond or outside the uterus. This effect may be "silent" or painful and can result in infertility.

endometrium The inner lining tissues of the uterus that respond to influences of estrogen and progesterone hormones.

equine estrogen A group of estrogens which are natural to horses, extracted from the urine of pregnant mares.

estradiol (E_2) The major active estrogen produced in humans.

estriol (E_3) A weakly estrogenic byproduct of estradiol metabolism, which is highest during pregnancy.

estrogen therapy Supplementing estrogen to relieve the symptoms of menopause.

estrone (E_1) A weak estrogen that is converted to estrone sulfate, which acts as a pool of estrone and can be converted as needed to the more active form of estrogen—estradiol.

fibroids   The common word for benign smooth muscle tumors or growths of the uterus, also referred to as myomata.

hysterectomy   Surgical removal of the uterus.

medroxy progesterone acetate (MPA)   A progestin used to treat menstrual disorders and to suppress the uterine lining in hormone replacement therapy, often in combination with estrogen.

menopause   The time when a woman can no longer get pregnant—one year after the final menstrual period and all the years that follow.

menstrual period/menses   The monthly flow of blood and cellular debris discarded from the uterus, which would have nourished an embryo had conception occurred. Menses begins at puberty and ends in menopause.

myomata   Benign tumor of smooth muscles, usually in the uterus (referred to as fibroids), often causing bleeding and sometimes pelvic or back pain.

myomectomy   Surgical removal of myoma (fibroids).

"natural aging"   Aging without the use of hormone supplementation.

norethindrone   A synthetic progestin used to oppose the effects of estrogen, typically provided through the skin or by mouth, paired with bioidentical estradiol.

opposed estrogen   The correct balance of estrogen with progesterone to prevent uterine cancer.

orgasm The highest point of sexual excitement, marked by strong feelings of pleasure and by vaginal contractions within the female and by ejaculation of semen from the male.

ovary Either of the paired female sexual glands in which oocytes (eggs) are formed, stored, and released at ovulation. The ovaries also produce estrogen and a certain amount of testosterone, and after monthly ovulation, releases progesterone.

pelvic floor The soft tissues supporting the bladder, urethra, vagina, cervix, and uterus, as well as the lower section of the colon, rectum, and anus. It is composed of both voluntary muscles (under your deliberate control) and involuntary muscles (guided by the nervous system).

perimenopause The transitional years preceding menopause, defined by irregular hormone patterns in the five to eight years before the final menstrual period. For example, a woman whose final menstrual period occurred at age 45 entered perimenopause at about age 37.

plant-based hormones Hormone products developed from plant molecules such as yam or soy. Bioidentical hormones are plant-derived and are exact copies of human hormones, whereas biosimilars are also derived from plants but imitate the formula of horse estrogen.

progestational effect A hormone effect similar to those of natural bioidentical progesterone. In menopause, it is used to oppose the stimulatory effects of estrogen to the uterine lining.

progesterone   A hormone in ovulating women, secreted by the ovaries after ovulation and by the placenta during pregnancy.

progestin   A steroid hormone prepared from plants that mimics some of the effects of natural progesterone, used in the prevention of endometrial hyperplasia.

steroid hormones   Hormones derived from cholesterol molecules, characterized by a specific chemical structure. It includes estrogens, progestagens, androgens, and two others. Vitamin D derivatives are a sixth closely related hormone system.

testosterone   A steroid hormone and the most potent naturally occurring androgen in women, which is formed by the ovaries and adrenal cortex.

transdermal delivery (trans meaning through and dermal meaning skin)   Providing a medication through the skin, such as bioidentical estradiol and testosterone, which are given through the skin via a cream, gel, patch, or spray.

transvaginal delivery   Providing a medication or supplement for absorption through the skin of the vagina via a tablet, suppository, cream, or ring.

urethra   The delicate tube that connects the urinary bladder to the outside of the body. The urethra is highly estrogen dependent and when estrogen levels fall, can become inflamed, develop scar tissue, and become a common source of pain with urination. These symptoms are often reversed with estrogen therapy.

uterine bleeding   Blood or liquefied menstrual products of endometrial cycling excreted through the cervix and vagina. In contrast to vaginal bleeding, it can also be caused by tears in the vaginal tissue due to severe atrophy or inflammation, or in rare cases due to cancer.

uterus (womb)   A muscular organ in the pelvis that nurtures the developing fetus. The uterine cavity is lined by endometrial tissue which grows in response to estrogen and thins out in response to progesterone.

vagina   A complex muscular chamber between the external vulva and the internal cervix (the neck of the uterus). It is comprised of a surface skin-like layer, a rich blood supply, moisture glands, elastin, collagen, and nerve fibers, all of which require estrogen.

Resources

Books

Check out the following list of books for more information on your health.

Self-Care

Agatston, Arthur, M.D., and Joseph Signorile, Ph.D. *The South Beach Diet Supercharged: FASTER Weight Loss and Better Health for Life*. St. Martin's Griffin, 2009.

———. *The South Beach Diet Quick & Easy Cookbook*. Rodale Books, 2005.

Anderson, Rodney, M.D., and David Wise, Ph.D. *A Headache in the Pelvis*, 5th Edition. National Center for Pelvic Pain, 2008.

Brand-Miller, Jennie, Ph.D., and others. *The New Glucose Revolution: The Authoritative Guide to the Glycemic Index*. Da Capo Press, 2006.

Butler, David, and Lorimer Moseley, M.D. *Explain Pain*. Orthopedic Physical Therapy Products, 2003.

Dean, Carolyn, M.D. *The Magnesium Miracle*. Ballantine Books, 2007.

Greene, Robert A., M.D., and Leah Feldon. *Perfect Balance*. Three Rivers Press, 2005.

Hanson, Rick, Ph.D., Jan Hanson, and Ricki Pollycove, M.D. *Mother Nurture: A Mother's Guide to Health in Body, Mind, and Intimate Relationships*. Penguin Books, 2002.

Parker-Pope, Tara. *The Hormone Decision*. Holtzbrink Publishers, 2007.

Pick, Marcelle, and Genevieve Morgan. *The Core Balance Diet: 4 Weeks to Boost Your Metabolism and Lose Weight for Good*. Hay House, 2009.

Shames, Richard, M.D., and Karilee Shames, Ph.D. *feeling fat, fuzzy, or frazzled?* Plume/Penguin Group, 2006.

Stein, Amy. *Heal Pelvic Pain*. McGraw-Hill, 2008.

Stewart, Elizabeth G., M.D., and Paula Spencer. *The V Book*. Bantam, 2002.

Mind-Body

Brizendine, Louann, M.D. *The Female Brain*. Broadway Books, 2006.

Farhi, Donna. *The Breathing Book: Good Health and Vitality Through Essential Breath Work*. Henry Holt, 1996.

Hanson, Rick, Ph.D., and Richard Mendius, M.D. *Buddha's Brain: The Practical Neuroscience of Happiness, Love & Wisdom*. New Harbinger, 2009.

Hulme, Janet. *Physiological Quieting* (audio CD).

Kabat-Zinn, Jon, Ph.D. *Mindfulness for Beginners*. (audio CD). Sounds True, 2006.

Kornfield, Jack. *A Path with Heart*. Bantam, 1993.

Lewis, Dennis. *The TAO of Natural Breathing for Health, Well-Being, and Inner Growth*. Mountain Wind Publishing, 1997.

Pert, Candice B., Ph.D. *Molecules of Emotion: The Science Behind Mind-Body Medicine*. Simon & Schuster Inc, 1997.

Smith, Jean, ed. *Breath Sweeps Mind*. Riverhead Books/Penguin Putnam, 1998.

Zukav, Gary. *The Seat of the Soul*. Fireside Books, 1989.

Lifestyle

Allen, David. *Getting Things Done: The Art of Stress-Free Productivity*. Penguin Books, 2001.

Bolen, Jean Shinoda, M.D. *Goddesses in Older Women: Archetypes in Women Over Fifty*. HarperCollins Publishers, 2001.

Jackson, Carole. *Color Me Beautiful*. Ballantine Books, 1987.

Kabat-Zinn, Jon, Ph.D. *Full Catastrophe Living: Using the Wisdom of Your Body and Mind to Face Stress, Pain, and Illness*. Dell Publishing, 2000.

Morgenstern, Julia. *SHED Your Stuff, Change Your Life: A Four-Step Guide to Getting Unstuck*. Fireside Books, 2009.

———. *Organizing from the Inside Out*. Holt Paperbacks, 2004.

Richardson, Cheryl. *The Art of Extreme Self-Care: Transform Your Life One Month at a Time*. Hay House, 2009.

———. *Take Time for Your Life*. Broadway Books, 1999.

Breast Health

Chan, David, M.D. *Breast Cancer: Real Questions, Real Answers*. Da Capo Press, 2006.

Kelly, Patricia, Ph.D. *Assess Your True Risk of Breast Cancer*. Henry Holt Company, LLC, 2000.

Peltason, Ruth. *I Am Not My Breast Cancer*. William Morrow, 2008.

Websites

The following are some helpful websites you can use to find out more information.

Menopause Information

health.nih.gov/category/WomensHealth. This page on women's health, within the larger NIH site, offers an extensive database of articles on every aspect of women's health, including lifestyle and prevention.

www.americanheart.org. Provides a download-able document on how to monitor your cholesterol, blood pressure, and weight.

www.cpmc.org/health/healthinfo. The site of the California Pacific Medical Center with links to an extensive database of articles on women's health, lifestyle, wellness, and numerous medical topics.

www.menopause.org. Site of the North American Menopause Society, a professional organization. The site includes a large consumer section with menopause information, referral lists, and links.

www.nia.nih.gov/HealthInformation. This National Institute on Aging site provides extensive publications (many free) and information.

Physical Therapy and Medical Conditions

www.ic-network.com. The Interstitial Cystitis Network (ICN), a resource for people who have been diagnosed with painful bladder syndrome (Interstitial Cystitis).

www.nva.org. The National Vulvodynia Association (NVA) site provides up-to-date information on the diagnosis of vulvodynia and related issues, including a free 24-page patient guide, available on request.

www.pelvicpain.org. The International Pelvic Pain Society (IPPS) covers topics related to pelvic pain with downloadable brochures and information on finding a provider.

www.womenshealthapta.org/plp/index.cfm. The Women's Health section of the website for the American Physical Therapy Association. This consumer-oriented site provides information and fact sheets on topics such as osteoporosis.

Index

I-J-K

L

M

Q-R